I am grateful to Grand Master Nan Hui-Jin,
and thank him for having written thirty two wonderful books,
which have helped me know my own culture even better.
I also thank the many Chinese qigong masters who have
unselfishly explored and passed on their valuable exercise forms
and experiences, such as Dr. Yan Xin
and Grand Master Tian Rei-Sheng.
And my thanks to the unselfish laws of the Chinese government
that all the Chinese ancient books are an open treasure
for humankind.

Copyright © 1996

ISBN 0-9652792-1-9

QIGONG ASSOCIATION OF AMERICA
27133 FOREST SPRINGS LANE
CORVALLIS, OR 97330
(541) 745-6310

All rights reserved. No part of this publication may be reproduced
or transmitted in any form or by any means, electronic or
mechanical, including photocopy without permission in writing
from the Qigong Association of America.

Printed in the United States of America.

Qi, The Treasure and Power of Your Body

BY YANLING L.JOHNSON

Copyright © Yanling L. Johnson September, 1995

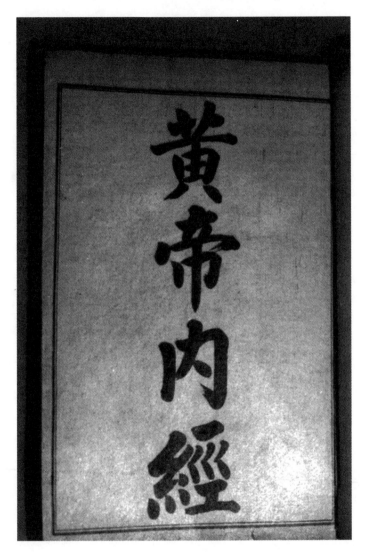

THE YELLOW EMPORER'S NEI JING;
WRITTEN 475 - 221 B.C.

By Yanling L. Johnson

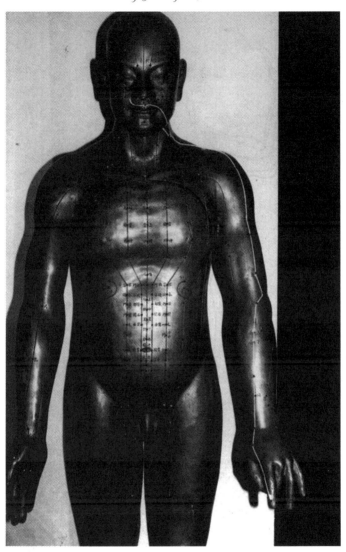

THE BRONZE ACUPUNCTURE FIGURE
MADE 1027 A.D.; HUMAN SIZE.

Table of Contents

Introduction

When I was a child, I saw the qigong masters perform: this was the beginning of my fascination with qigong. For twenty-two years I taught at the high school level, both in China and the United States. While teaching, qigong was only as a method to relax my mind. But there is much more to the advantages of qigong.

Qigong, acupuncture, and herbs have not been accepted by contemporary Western medicine and Western science. This is sad for mankind because these treatment methods have worked for people for thousands of years.

In 1990 I quit teaching to work on qigong and writing. My interests led me to help with the translation of a few of many types of qigong in 1991. Later, with the aid of friends, I helped establish The Qigong Association of America and organize numerous workshops. We discovered a wonderful qigong teacher, Professor Chen Huixian, who presently teaches at the Oregon College of Oriental Medicine.

This book is based upon the practices of some well-known Grand Masters, as well as what I have learned through my own experiences. I wish to express great respect and thanks to Dr. Nan Huai-jin, who has written thirty-two wonderful books, and Dr. Yan Xin. I have met neither, but have learned a lot from both. I hope to someday meet them, to consult and learn more from them; an even greater wish is to be able to translate more of the wisdom found in the Chinese culture, and to share these treasures of mankind with you. I'll try my best.

What is Tao? What is Qigong?

CHAPTER 1

Qigong is an advanced form of healing, though in many ways it is more than healing. Its history begins at least five thousand years ago. It is an Eastern science that modern Western science cannot yet explain. Qigong is the best, most inexpensive doctor anyone can afford.

Western culture often sees Taoism and Buddhism simply as religions. But to the millions of people who practice them, they are not only religions; they are forms of advanced science and are ultimately valuable in helping people attain tao.

What is tao? You have undoubtedly seen the yin/yang symbols, currently popular in some Western fashions. In the well known book *I Ching*, it said the yin and yang are tao. Constant change, following the natural discipline of the universe, is tao. Confucius explained: "To see its function by using it is tao."

Dr. Nan Hui-jin called the *I Ching* a "book of the universe". According to the *I Ching*, death and birth are two sides of yin and yang, both in tao. But the author of the *I Ching* did not dwell on the word "death". He focused on "birth" and "growth" to describe our world. Like the sun, life rises and falls, moving in a circle day after day. There is always change, always a new future. Bad always follows the good, which always follows bad.

Tao is about the universe, including all the stars and the space in between. It is about how the earth was formed–according to the universe's natural ways.

Tao is also a way to help humans to recognize themselves and to explore their latent power, the potential that

8

we were born with but have lost sight of.

Where is tao? It is everywhere. But don't try to look for it, you will not find it: it is inside yourself. It can not be less or more. You can not make it grow or die. What you need to do is to know yourself. This is studying tao. This is starting to work on qigong.

Why do people do tai chi and meditation? For health, for longevity? Or for spiritual purposes? The famous ancient scholars and Grand Masters – Lao Tzu and the Lord Buddha – and many contemporary Chinese scholars have answered "yes" to all of these purposes. There is a possibility that human life can be extended indefinitely (many cultures have faith that a human's spirit never dies). Qigong may be a part of the way.

How do we begin? Buddha told his students that he had provided them the boat to cross the river; as soon as they crossed the river they were on their own and it would be best not to carry the boat on their backs during their journey. Confucius gave ten of his students ten different answers to the same one question. Why? We all need to think about it. Hopefully the following chapters can help you in some way.

How to Start

CHAPTER 2

Simply put, a qigong learner should be a decent person. You should have a strong heart and a desire to promote good, not evil. Perhaps you have not always been a person of integrity. Perhaps you have a criminal record, or carry with you painful memories of hurtful actions you have done. If you are determined to change, and not harm others again, you can start learning qigong.

You should begin by learning first about qi and about qigong.

Qi (pronounced as "chi") is everywhere. It is not the same as tao, which is like the spiritual property of everything. Nor is it the same as air or water, which are physical things you can see and feel. It is a sort of energy. All living things absorb and release qi all the time, just like the nose and mouth and pores in the skin breathe in oxygen and drive out waste. Everyone of us already has this ability. Some people possess more in utilizing qi than others. Qigong helps to improve this ability, and develop this power to explore the many potential abilities you were born with. Bill Moyers' wonderful program *Healing in the Mind* showed some great examples of the powers humans can obtain. Scientists have done research on qi and qigong for years and have proved much of it, although they often find it difficult to explain.

Your qi powers can be developed by working on them. Developing a moral balance will help you improve your ability to learn and reach your greatest potential. To be kind to the world, to love, to help, to forgive, and to have a strong heart: these are all important, so you will be in the most relaxed, carefree state. This is the best condition for your body to absorb and send qi. And it is also the way to start working on attaining the tao.

After you begin to pursue qigong, reading and studying more, you will find in the world more pleasure and happiness. And there will be much more beyond that. There are many types of qigong. There are moving forms, meditation forms and others. Well-known Grand Qigong Master Dr. Yan Xin said there are 36,000 Taoist and 84,000 Buddhist types of qigong. It would be a tremendous work to learn them all. It may also be unnecessary. Sure, by learning more than one, you understand qi and qigong better. But for a beginner, you must choose one type to start with.

Start with a moving exercise first. It will help open up the blockages and soothe the qi channels of the body (for the channels will not be all open yet) and prepare you for learning more types, including the advanced gong – meditation. It is better to exercise the moving form for at least three months. Then you can learn meditation.

What is Qi?

CHAPTER 3

Some define qi as "vital energy" but it is actually more than that though Qi and qigong are not all powerful and cannot purify some people's lives. For most people, however, they can lead to many benefits.

The first chapter of the Chinese classic of medical works, the Yellow Emperor's *Nei Jing*, starts with qigong and how qi treats diseases. The Yellow Emperor described the qi channels in the human body and said that a good doctor should treat "the future diseases", the invisible illnesses, the sicknesses with no symptoms at all. This skill would require the power of qigong.

According to Dr. Yan Xin's study, two thirds of the *Nei Jing* volumes utilize qigong. The other third focuses on herbs, but continues to relate to qigong in one way or another.

In 1990 the Chinese government's High-Energy Physics Institute began calling together and well-known qigong masters. These masters were asked to repeatedly perform specific qi research experiments. Some of the astonishing results were labeled "top secret". The top Chinese officials were apprehensive about releasing them to the world. As one example of their findings, the qigong masters were able to change the molecular structure of higher elements.

These scientists have proven that qi does exist, and that it is a kind of physical entity. It can change the nature of the food that people eat (for example, change the structure of glucose) so as to strengthen their immune system. It can penetrate several-thousand-volts;

it can generate its own voltage. It can also stimulate the growth of germs or of a virus. It can change bone structure: aged people who practice qigong can reduce and eliminate bone problems. It possesses a power that modern high-tech instruments do not.

Qigong will help strengthen the qi and help people become healthier. Qigong stimulates blood and bodily fluid circulation, smoothing the blockages inside the body. Qi is the only doctor that treats each individual differently; it is the only one that can find its way and follow its inclinations inside your body, to seek and attack diseases; it is the only one that is able to find the hidden diseases that modern instruments and most doctors cannot see. And it is the only one that can change the structure of cancer cells and cure certain types of cancer – this has been proven through the work and experiments of qigong masters done at the Chinese Navy General Hospital.

Qi is not at all like chemotherapy, the treatment that kills cancer cells and at the same time gradually kills the patient. Qi kills the viruses chemicals can't. Some doctors are able to send qi through the needles they use to treat patients. (They do not need alcohol to clean the needles and have been known to insert them directly through the patient's clothing. When checked, they are even cleaner than needles sterilized with alcohol.)

Qi is the greatest psychotherapist. People who practice it and understand it become well adjusted, their innermost beings become calm and satisfied.

No modern Western instruments seem to be able to prove what qi, and the qi channels, exactly are. Chinese researchers have used some instruments to show that there is light sparkling in the channels and in the main acupoints. These lights are not invisible to all people, however.

Qigong can not only strengthen your energy (the qi), but can help you discover your potential ability as it can help you regain the powers hidden with in your subconscious.

What are Jing, Qi, and Shen?

CHAPTER 4

I have seen people wearing T-shirts with the three characters, jing, qi, and shen, on them. I often wonder whether they know much about these three important words, their power or how they are the essence of the qigong culture.

The ancient Chinese character "qi" is formed by two parts, "none" and "fire". In other words, if a person has no fire-like desires, no longing, no worry, no desire, no recklessness to disturb the mind, it is qi. To maintain a peaceful, calm, relaxed mind is qi.

Taoism says if a person truly and fully masters jing, qi, and shen, then he or she will become immortal.

The three words do not mean something material, nor physical. They are inside you. They are also in the universe. But as Confucius said, "jing qi" condenses and forms our material, physical world. When we are living, the shen is inside us. When we die, our shen changes and goes to another world.

Let's discuss the three words separately.

Qi does not just mean breathing, but breathing naturally, deeply, down to the lower stomach at first, later breathing through the navel and eventually merging yourself into the natural world as an organic whole. You will feel the warmth that begins from the lower dan tian, a bodily focus centered in the abdomen, near the navel.

Jing means a peaceful, calm mind and a cool, sweet, refreshing feeling of vitality. You will feel it gradually, little by little, as it starts from the middle channel in the front of the body. It later spreads all over the body, reach-

15

ing the head. Then you will feel enlightened. Do not be reluctant to wonderful images and visions: let them be. You will feel the saliva you produce tastes sweet and refreshing. Swallow it all at once, sending it down into the lower dan tian.

Shen is the spirit guide. It means the mind is free from the material world. It is a feeling that only you can feel. It is your true heart, a heart of tao. No matter how deep the meditation you are in, that little shen – the little light, your conscious – is always above your head with you and can guide you back whenever you want to finish the qigong.

Why Virtue is Important in Learning Qigong

CHAPTER 5

The I Ching said, "The natural world owns the wealth. It created everything, not by taking but by giving." To give, then, is a virtue. The I Ching described virtue as "making progress day after day". Dr. Nan Hui-jin explains this as "learning and improving every day. There is only tomorrow. Today is gone. Do not focus on yesterday; it is gone - it is gone. Do not live in the past."

Human energy is of two kinds: bad or good, negative or positive. Like a knife, it can save lives but it can also kill. When you give love, when you care, the same kind of energy is returned. When you respect and help people, you feel peaceful inside: you are developing a positive energy and giving your body a positive message. When Jesus was bleeding on the cross and dying, he was selflessly atoning for the world. He prayed for the world, not for himself. What an extraordinary heart! If we can adopt that kind of heart, we can learn qigong much more quickly and correctly.

Respecting our elders is not just virtuous, but useful. It is an important way of learning. Elderly people have experience and wisdom that young people do not. By learning from their wisdom, we can avoid wasting time and energy unnecessarily. We can do more of the things we want. To respect them will only benefit you. Someday you will become old, and you will understand. And, yes, respecting older people is also part of virtue - they have lived their share and deserve your respect.

Do not steal, do not lie, do not take part in other

17

bad acts. Be good to all living things. Any negative or guilty feelings will disturb qi. Try to participate in as many good deeds as you can. All these positive feelings will help you make progress in learning qigong. In China, some Grand Masters require their students serve society before studying qigong.

No one is born a bigot, a bully or a bad person. Our body fills up like a gold mine, as the Lord Buddha told his people. Impurities develop as we grow. "In order to enjoy the gold, you have to extract and purify it from the ore." This "gold" has been inside you since you were born; it depends only on you whether you want to extract and purify it. Or, as Buddha told us, you were born a buddha, but later were made squalid and unclean by the material world. As the nature of gold will never change, so your nature will never change. If you start working on it now, you can help the "real you" come back. And qigong can help you purify your body.

But first of all, you should purify your mind. The first important thing in learning qigong well is to work on yourself, to be a good person. Keep this thought – "I am a good person" – in your mind at all times, and take action to maintain this. Keep it solidly in your mind, as the way you miss your loved ones when they are away. You'll improve your qigong quickly.

Before Starting

CHAPTER 6

First of all, before you start exercising qigong, think of something that makes you happy. You should try to smile 24 hours a day in your heart. Focus for a moment on something pleasant just before you exercise.

Whenever you do qigong, you will always keep the tip of your tongue up touching the maxilla slightly, keeping your mouth slightly closed. The maxilla is the point on the roof of your mouth, just behind the front teeth.

You will also learn to understand different qigong phrases. "To close your eyes" means to keep the outside world from disturbing you, to remain calm and peaceful, to forget physical sensations. If your mind is unable to be in such a state, just physically closing your eyes will not help. Ultimately you will be able to keep your eyes open but still remain in such a state.

"To relax" means to relieve tension from both the body and the mind. The three main parts of your body to relax are your neck, your waist and your lower stomach.

"To follow the steps strictly" does mean strictly in the sense with which you are familiar. Each movement is designed for a reason. It is not only a physical exercise but, more importantly, is a movement to guide the qi to flow along the proper channels. You'll understand it better after you exercise for a time (maybe a long time) and the qi movement becomes more obvious. At first, you may not strongly feel the flow of qi. It depends on the individual. It will also depend on how you do your qigong.

Another thing you need to know is that if one type of qigong does not work for you after a long time, some-

19

thing may be wrong with the way you are doing it. It may be the hour, the place or the environment.

If it ends up being none of these things, only then should you consider another type of qigong. Do not change qigong types frequently - that will certainly not do you good. Different individuals make different progress. More sensitive people may make better progress, for example.

If some part of your body feels more sensitive to qi than other parts, pay more attention to it. Focus on where you feel more sensitive.

You can gain a great deal from exercising during the time of the traditional festivals. At these times many people meet, including the ancestors, and there is a lot positive energy. The energy of ancient messages from the festivals of long ago may be sensed and shared. The positive energy during festivals will benefit you more, and you may receive some of the messages and become wiser and stronger.

If you experience problems, remember that it is not qigong that is causing them. Qigong does not cause problems, you must question whether or not you are not doing it properly.

Choosing a Moving Form First

CHAPTER 7

There are so many types of qigong. It is important to begin with only one type first. Stick to that type of qigong and do it continuously, every day. If you lack perseverance, it is like driving a car but continually turning off the engine. You will make little progress, and waste your time and energy. The moving form helps move the qi, helps open the blockages, calms the mind and exercises the body.

Although you have to follow the steps strictly, don't follow them in a mechanical manner. Pay attention to how you feel about each movement, as well as how you feel about the time and place you are exercising. Adjust if it feels uncomfortable. After you have mastered the type of gong that you have learned, try to learn more about qigong in general. Observe yourself and the changes you have experienced, and try to find the most effective movement for you. If you want to make more progress and learn more about qigong, you will move on to more forms and different types throughout your life. And you will learn from whomever is better than you.

Meditation

CHAPTER 8

Meditation is a process of changing yin into yang.

To meditate is not simply to "empty your mind". No one can truly empty his or her mind. Thoughts do come into your mind when you are meditating. This is normal. You don't force them out: that is the wrong way to meditate. If you were able to force yourself to empty your mind successfully and continued doing this for a long time, let's say for years, you might gain some kind of power. But you would not attain tao. Instead you would become a person prone to outrageousness or without feelings! That should not be your goal.

How do you perform meditation?

First, do it sincerely. Have faith. Meditate on an empty stomach; it will help clean the body. And relax. The proper way is to let each thought come, then let it go. Before the second thought comes, try to make the emptiness last a bit longer. When the second thought comes, let it come, and let it go. Before the third one comes, try to make the space last as long as you can, until the fourth thought comes, and so on. If you keep doing meditation in the right way, someday you will be able to maintain a stable, peaceful, calm-minded state. That is the beginning of success.

If your mind is disturbed by something, "suit the remedy to the cause" and find out the exact reason. Is it caused by some physical stimulus? Qi channel blockage (for example, you become angry easily)? The wrong food? Poor nutrition?

For example, when a person's nutrition is weak, qi

may go through the Yu Zhen points. The person may either get red eyes or a symptom like cataracts. After continued meditation, and an improvement in nutrition, the symptoms will go away.

Sometimes the qi is not regulated well; it may go the wrong way and adversely affect the organs. Or your shen may be shocked; you may be hurt by someone or something, so you are in low spirits. You must seek out the cause and reason out a solution.

Also, many of our worries and bad premonitions are just illusions. These unreal images come from your own mind. Ignore them.

There are many ways to meditate; Dr. Yan Xin said there are 118 types of meditation. People mainly do the standing, sitting or lying forms. But the basic type, and also the most advanced type, is the sitting posture. Of course, sitting meditation also has many variations. The best way is to sit on a pad or pillow with your legs crossed.

Breath counting is a common and effective way to calm the mind. Like the many other ways, it is to use the counting to get rid of your troubled thoughts. However, people with lower blood pressure or who are weak should count inhales only. Stronger, average people or those with higher blood pressure should count exhales. Count from one to ten, repeat again, until your breathing becomes soft and slow, and you can stop counting.

Remember to try to maintain a peaceful, calm mind, and remain aware of what you are learning, no matter where you are, what time it is, whatever you are doing. It is all right to be upset, or overjoyed, or sad, or angry. But let go of these emotions quickly and don't indulge in them. If you can master this, you will be in a state of meditation all the time.

Think about qigong all day long. This is like keeping the camp fire burning. Grand Master Yan Xin suggested to busy people that before they start work, they focus their minds on the heart for a minute, even for just a half minute or less. You can do this also when shifting from one task to another, and at the end of the work day as well. Of course, properly you should always "end the gong" when finishing the one task and going on to another. All you need to do is visualize all the good qi returning to your lower dan tian.

Do qigong all the time, everyday, and the qi campfire will not die; you will be able to rekindle the qi at any time, in an instant.

Dr. Nan Huai-jin once told one of his students to think of himself as a ten-year-old boy who just woke up on a spring morning. He told him to visualize lying in bed, relaxed, too lazy to move, but not drowsy. That moment describes the state to be in when you are doing meditation.

Now, don't be wishing you would reach a certain higher level or gain a certain power. Just forget it, because your desire will be a burden on your mind and will not set your mind free. It will hamper your ability to make progress.

What are the tangible benefits of meditation?

It is easy to improve your health if you do qigong continuously. But it takes both time and comprehension to enter the true meditation state. After a long time, if you have been doing it the right way, you will learn to enter that state - you will feel your whole body is weightless, and soft as a baby, as if you can float on air. You will feel a flow of coolness, a pleasant feeling flowing from the top of your head and flowing all way down to the bottom of your feet.

The flow may also start from the bottom of your feet and travel up to the top of your head. This kind is more desirable. The flow that starts from the head will wane easily, but not the flow that starts from the bottom of your feet. But since you can not wish for it, nor guide it, do not try. Just accept. Let it be as it is.

If you practice meditation regularly, don't ever panic, no matter what happens - you may hear a voice talking to you, or unexpectedly see a loved one whom you are missing appear in front of you, or suddenly find a book in your pocket that did not belong to you. Just be yourself, remain calm, so you will not lose the power you might have gained, the power that is causing these surprising events.

Through meditation, you can reach a high level, higher lever, and higher....

You may have heard of the sixth sense. But according to the qigong theory, you have even more than the sixth sense. What more is there? How will you feel if you experience it? Only by yourself, by continuously doing qigong, may you experience it, and only you yourself can be responsible for it.

There are people who have learned to use more than their five common senses. Both Dr. Nan Huai-jin and Dr. Yan Xin, as well as other Grand Masters, ensure us that there are sixth, seventh, eighth senses – call them super power senses – and they can be used. It sounds inconceivable, but it is true. Chinese scientists have experienced some.

A few well-known Chinese journalists have interviewed some of those Grand Masters, and have experienced their powers – powers like you have seen only in the movies, the stories of fantasy.

This may sound very exciting and empowering. But remember: do not long for it. Then it will never happen.

Cautions

CHAPTER 9

Why can mushrooms grow by themselves on one piece of wood? There are no "germs" to help them grow. They grow themselves. Similarly, you grow your own germ – diseases. Taoism says that overworking yourself physically will kill you, and thinking too much will change your own nature. Only when these two work together harmoniously will a person stay healthy. In this way, only qigong can help you.

So many people practice qigong. There are many types of qigong and there are many teachers. There is also a growing number of qigong video tapes made and books written. It is unwise to learn qigong only from a tape or from a book. The best way is to learn from a qualified teacher. When you learn and practice qigong, you have to learn some knowledge first. The following is something that a qigong learner needs to know.

1. Never move against the flow of the natural world: the season, the temperature, the geography, etc. The human body is affected by the natural world. Always adapt yourself to the changes in the environment. Spring and summer are full of yang energy, while autumn and winter are the yin seasons. During the strong yang seasons, be careful to nurture and store yin energy. During the yin seasons nurture and store yang.

2. Do not rage. Anger harms the yin energy in your body and harms the liver. Do not indulge in grief; it harms the yang energy in your body and also your kidneys. Al-

ways try to maintain a balance of yin and yang.

3. Do not exercise during storms or strong winds, or in too hot or too cold an environment. Harmonize with the atmosphere.

4. Do not exercise in polluted or smoky areas. While helping to conserve energy, qigong stimulates and supplies the material base of the body - the qi. When exercising qigong, large amounts of air will be inhaled and exhaled. If the air around you causes coughing, shortness of breath, a stuffy chest, and dizziness, it will retard your progress and harm you.

5. People who have rheumatism or heart conditions related to dampness should not exercise near waterfalls, rivers, the ocean or in damp, cold caves.

6. Do not exercise against the wind. Keep warm and dry.

7. Do not exercise near stagnant water because it may give off harmful vapors.

8. While it is bad to exercise near harmful plants, many are helpful. The volatile elements of the cypress and fir trees can destroy some unwanted germs and even virus. They are the best trees for qigong exercisers.
Trees like eucalyptus, cassia, clove, lemon, and lime provide beneficial aromas and oils that clean the air. Banyan helps bring up the qi, and is good for people who have low blood pressure or those who lack qi. But those with high blood pressure should abstain. Volatile sub-

stances given off by cypress and fir trees are good for those who have liver, lung, kidney, or gallbladder problems. The Chinese parasol tree and camphor tree are good for those with heart problems. Willow benefits those with stomach problems. All tea plants, orange trees, and bay trees are good.

But yulan magnolia, longan, the Chinese scholar tree, peach, plum, oak, oleander, and other sensitive plants may cause some people dizziness, a stuffy chest, or shortness of breath, so some people should avoided doing qigong near them.

9. Do not exercise in noisy places if you have not prepared yourself well. Introverted people will excel under a clear starry sky and a bright moon between midnight and two a.m. Sanguine people should choose daytime where the scenery is pleasant.

10. Do not exercise when the air in the room is not fresh. Cactus and basket plants help freshen the air. The two color basket ("spider") plants are best and are said to be more effective than air filters.

11. Do not use the mind too much or breathe irregularly while practicing qigong. Relax the mind, turn inward. Always breathe in and out slowly, naturally, deeply and evenly.

12. Beginners should not attempt to modify the style of qigong they were taught. Stick to the teachings and do the exercises constantly, regularly, and consistently. Without proper knowledge, practicing different styles of qigong at the same time may cause problems.

For example, you may be focusing on one channel, while your body movements are guiding qi along another.

13. Practicing qigong is not only exercise; it is also the development of a transcending moral character. Only by being a virtuous person can one learn qigong well and eventually reach a higher level.

14. Do not believe in quick easy shortcuts.

15. Do not give thought to personal gains or losses, nor be too concerned about trifles. Be calm.

16. Do not remain undecided and of two minds when learning qigong. Qigong is a process, not a miracle.

17. Do not overtax yourself, or squander energy by seeking fame and wealth.

18. Do not follow any sounds or pictures that come into the mind as you practice qigong. There is no need to be alarmed by these visions, but you must keep calm and be detached. Do not try to figure out what they mean. Think instead that they have nothing to do with you. Do not wish that you could see or hear them again.

19. Do not be in a hurry to use the power you have gained. Use the power the little as you can. It costs you your energy to use it. When you are able to use it, do so in small amounts so you will not feel tired afterwards, so you do not exhaust your energy. Only when you have learned to protect and conserve yourself will you be able to help others.

20. Do not accept troubling messages while exercising. Do not fear that you might have a disease. Put your mind onto something else.

21. Do not give up when you feel impatient or irritable. When you feel it, stop and wait until you calm down. It indicates your body has problems and is in the process of healing. But also it might be a time when you are gaining some special power. Do some deep breathing, make some movements, make some sounds. When you are calm, continue the exercise. If you are unable to become calm, end the exercise. Impatience within the family may pass on to you and you may pass it on to the group. When one member of the family exercises it can benefit the entire family.

22. It is normal to feel some pain. It may be you are healing yourself or you are healing someone in your family. This may happen to the very sensitive exerciser. When you feel anger and want to cry or yell, do not control these feelings. Do not encourage them; rather, let yourself release them naturally.

23. Do not worry if you sleep less than usual, or have times of sleeplessness, as long as you continue to feel energetic. Keep exercising. However, if you must sleep, focus your mind on the bottom of your feet. Visualize lights circling at the bottom of your feet, from 36 to 49 times. Or imagine the light circling your navel. This will help you sleep.

To be sleepless and still energetic is a sign of health and is a result of practicing qigong. To become tired as a result of sleeplessness may indicate sickness.

24. When doing standing meditation spontaneous movements may happen, especially to those who have health problems. Do not be alarmed by large scale, spontaneous movements. They are a good sign that the qi is working on a blockage inside your body. Do no try to control them. Thinking of a good thought such as, "My lungs will get stronger." Then let it go and relax. And to start with a pleasant thought before you start doing meditation can avoid violent movement. However, doing it for too long of a time and with too violent movements can drain the qi. Better doing it for no more than an hour. It will help if you tell yourself that your movements are going to be gentle before you start.

25. Do not panic if you cannot stop your spontaneous movements. Should they become violent, think of yourself and the safety of others, such as "Do not hurt myself or other people, nor damage property." Change your gestures, sit or lie down, and concentrate on guiding the movements gently, and little by little so they slow down. Others may use words to slow the exerciser's movements. Before you begin exercising tell yourself that you are a good person and able to do anything you really want to do. It will help to avoid violent movements.

26. After practicing qigong for a long time, some things may begin to change. You may not want to eat. If you are still energetic it is fine and may be considered a good sign. Do not force yourself to eat. Eat when you are hungry; drink when you are thirsty.

27. Having good habits helps maintain yourself in good health. Preventing disease is more important than

treating disease. Such as: comb your hair often; avoid sharp winds on the back of your head and neck; do not make love when drunk; soak your feet in warm water regularly; massage the bottom of your feet before going to bed; eat healthy food; never overeat in the evening; eat less meat and more vegetables, etc.

28. Do not seek out more complicated forms of qigong. More complex types are not necessarily better. It can be as simple as this: during the day focus your mind on the navel; after dusk focus the mind on the top of the head (but not when you are too hungry or too full); rub your palms until they are hot, then put them over the navel; at night put your tongue on the upper maxilla. These simple things are qigong, too.

29. Do not disrupt your biological clock. For example, the ability of the liver to remove toxins is lower in summer and higher in winter. So be more careful about what you eat in summer. Live your life with regularity.

30. Do not sleep or attempt to perform sitting meditation on a soft bed.

31. Keep the air fresh when you exercise qigong inside the house. But do not let air blow directly on your body; keep at least three feet away from open windows.

32. Do not use a high pillow. It should not be higher than your shoulder when lying down.

33. Use cotton fabric bedding.

34. Sleep on your side, rather than sleeping on your back.

35. Do not sleep in a draft. Do not sleep with your mouth open. Empty yourself before going to bed.

36. Winter is the season when it is easier to catch a cold. Do not exercise to a sweat out of doors or stay outside for too long. It may harm the kidney qi. Eat food to nourish your yang: lamb, chicken, or beef in winter. Also take some herb tonic, such as ginseng, but only enough for your own body's needs. (For people whose yang energy is very strong, ginseng is not good.)

37. Eat more fruit and less sugar. Use more vinegar and less salt. Salty foods may harm the kidneys. Do not eat one particular kind of food for too long; eat a wide variety of foods.

38. Clean your teeth often. To brush the teeth before going to bed is more important than in the morning. Chewing your food thoroughly is not just good for digestion, but also is an exercise for your teeth. Before you get up, "knock" your teeth to exercise them.

39. All diseases relate to the organs; organs relate to the moods and conversely moods affect the organs. Too much worry, anger, upset, grief, or nervousness can interfere with the smooth flow of qi and blood and in this way unbalance the functioning of the organs. Try always to maintain a peaceful mood.

40. The nature of each person is different. Part of

your nature is in you from birth, part is acquired. There are five basic personalities:

a.) those who are optimistic but impatient; they should try to enjoy the natural world more, eat less spicy food, and practice a quiet qigong style.

b.) those who worry much, are introverted and timid, and are self-abasing and not too happy much of the time; they may drink a little wine daily and eat chenpi (dried tangerine skin) and shangzha rice soup often and use some herbs to soothe the liver and to release liver bad qi.

c.) those who are optimistic, carefree, resourceful, and calm and like to socialize; they should eat light and practice quiet type of qigong.

d.) those who are quiet, calm, honest, and sincere, and who do not talk much; they should lead a regular life, be cautious about drinking wine and eating spicy foods, relax more, seek entertainment, and practice quiet type of qigong.

e.) those who change easily, and are narrow-minded, jealous, and frivolous; they should become involved in doing good deeds and choosing nice people as friends. They should think before taking action or speaking, and should practice quiet type of qigong.
All of these types may shift from one to the other over time.

41. Choose a place where qigong masters have practiced would be even better because it conveys positive mes-

sages and has a lingering positive atmosphere.

42. Do not make any noise breathing in and out while doing meditation. Do not breathe in a broken way; keep it smooth, continuous and soft.

43. Do not lower your head or allow a frisky "monkey mind" during meditation. Calm the mind slowly. If you should try to calm the mind too quickly you might feel "head heavy" or experience some chest pain. Just relax the mind and imagine the qi going down your middle channel. Sometimes when your mind is not on meditation your body may lean to the side and saliva will drool out of the corner of your mouth. Then you must focus your mind quickly and gently on meditation.

44. Five things will have adverse effects on the results of meditation:

a.) greed

b.) thoughts of revenge, anger or hatred

c.) sleeping

d.) regrets about something in the past

e.) doubting your ability to meditate, doubting your teacher, or doubting the meditation method.

45. Do not lose your calm when a disturbance occurs. Quickly recall the mood and the feeling before the disturbance happened. Your mind will quickly readjust

when the disturbance is resolved. Otherwise, sudden noises may disrupt the mind. Other people may help the distraught one by giving some honey or fruit to eat and telling him to imagine a mirror in front of him and friends and family looking at him.

46. Do not focus the mind on one position all the time while meditating. For example, do not focus only on the upper body. A single focus might result in a trance-like or depressed state. If the mind focuses on the lower body parts for extremely long periods of time, one might feel body-heavy or one may even faint.

47. Do not delay treatment if the wrong exercise causes trouble. First find the cause, then treat it with proper breathing.

If the trouble is caused by an improper sitting posture, it may be sending qi into the top of the head. Treat this by sending qi down along the spine, pausing at each joint, and gradually sending qi down into the tail joint. Repeat several times to resolve the problem.

If the trouble is caused by breathing, first correct your method of breathing. Then, after qi is breathed in, hold it for a while, visualizing qi from the top of the head spreading into the entire body, into the four limbs, and spreading out to cover the skin. This exercise, continued for a long time, will make your skin smooth and your joints dexterous and quick.

48. If you meditate by counting your breathing, but do it in the wrong way, your breathing pattern will be harmed. To correct the problem, loosen your clothing, contract qi with the mouth closed, and send the qi up to

the top of the head, then down again repeating until your breathing is calm and normal.

49. If you are feeling stuffy and short of breath, breathe out with a "xu-" sound, then breathe in through the nose sending qi over all the body. Focus the mind on the two palms and soon you will feel fine.

50. If it feels as if qi is stuck in the upper chest and the stomach feels bloated, loosen the clothing and adjust your breathing. Breathe out long and breathe in short ten times.

51. If a problem is caused by breathing in and out too quickly, first relax the mind; if you are feeling top heavy, fix the mind on the navel; if the opposite, fix the mind on the top of the nose, or in the middle between the eyebrows.

52. If the problem is a headache, breathe in through the nose and slowly out through the mouth. At the same time imagine the headache is gone.

53. If, while sitting in meditation, the mouth relaxes to one side, let the mind follow to the same side. The mouth will center itself normally.

54. If you feel your limbs are weak, possibly caused by the wrong meditation, visualize qi moving to fill your four limbs.

55. If the five organs feel bloated, use your mind to take qi out the bottom of your feet and down into the

earth while breathing out.

56. Improper breathing may cause coughing. Just before you are going to cough, stifle it; breathe out three times, then focus your mind on your chest.

57. If, after sitting meditation, you feel your stomach is full of gas, breathe in slowly through the nose, then out again slowly. Visualize the bloated qi being breathed out. If you feel your stomach is full of hard things, lie on your back, stretch out your arms and legs, and use your hands to gently massage your stomach 10 to 15 times; "burp" out the gas.

58. When doing sitting meditation, your back should not be against the back of the chair as it will affect the smooth movement of the qi.

59. When doing sitting meditation, if the mind is at the lower dan tian and you begin to feel the qi, then the mind should not focus on the lower dan tian and let the qi move by itself. Forget yourself and the world. If your mind is on another point, after you feel the movement of the qi, let it go naturally; do not follow after it; instead forget the world and yourself.

60. When sitting meditation, spontaneous movement better not happen. If it happens, tell your body, "Spontaneous movement is not appropriate in meditation," and thereby control yourself. If this does not stop the movement, end the meditation. Perform qigong exercises until the channels are cleared; then return to the meditation.

61. It is not good to sleep while doing sitting meditation. If you fall asleep, find out the reason. If fatigue is caused by too much sex, you may do the double returning qi three times. The person who is not suited to meditation should stop.

62. As you go to sleep, breathing in and visualizing qi entering the bottom of your feet will benefit your health. Breathe deeply through the nose often, sending qi throughout the whole body, then slowly close the mouth and move the qi from the top of the head and progressing downward. This also benefits health.

63. When you go to the bathroom to eliminate waste, focus on sending any bad qi out with it. This is also good for treating diseases.

64. Do not tell others what you see during meditation or what improvements you have made.

65. When meditating, sometimes your sexual desire may suddenly become strong. To release may result in emission and you would lose what you have gained from the meditation. One of the best way is to focus on the meditation and try to let the desire go naturally if you can.

66. Remain in harmony with the four seasons. In the spring, get up early and do not eat too much sour food. Sour food can harm the spleen. Increase your outdoor exercise, but not in the wind. While facing south tap the teeth together three times.

In summer sleep well at night and get up early. Do

not lie in a damp place. Keep your clothing dry. Do not eat too much cold food; instead add some spicy food to your diet. Avoid winds.

In autumn go to bed early and get up early. Eat less spicy food and more sour food. Sesame is good. Avoid cold drinks; avoid damp clothing.

In winter go to bed early and get up late. Do not wear clothing that is too warm. Do not stand close to the fire too often. Drink a little wine each day. Reduce the amount of sour food and add some bitter food to your diet. Face north when you meditate. Imagine that the north star is giving out black qi directly into your mouth and sending it directly to the kidneys.

67. Do not eat at irregular times or eat food that is too hot or too cold, or too greasy. Do not eat too much at one meal. This may harm the organs.

68. Do not ignore healthy food; a good diet is better than medicine. Foods also exert mutual promotion and restraint between each other. With certain diseases one should avoid certain foods. Patients who have sores or skin ulcers should not eat seafood, heads of chickens, pork, beef, or lamb. Nor should they use onion, ginger, hot pepper, or wine. While taking ginseng do not eat radish. Eat more vegetables and fruit. Eat the right foods according to the four seasons.

69. Mind proper nutrition. Elderly people should eat a suitable amount of fruit. Some fruits are not good for the elderly because they should not eat too much: such as banana, apple, orange, and grape. Eat them, but in moderation.

70. During qigong exercise it is better not to drink. Do not take vitamin supplements without guidance. Regular healthy meals are better than vitamin supplements.

71. Stop smoking. The nicotine in the smoke is poisonous and addictive. Qigong works to rid the body of toxins. Why pump them back in? Alcohol and wine are poison, unless they are used in a proper way. Rheumatism patients may drink a little herbal wine daily.

72. Different disease conditions require different foods. Different foods have different functions. A local acupuncturist should be able to answer your specific questions.

73. Qigong exercisers should be very selective about what they eat.

74. Do not cook herbs in an iron pot. It may lessen the benefits and even produce a toxin.

75. Sick exercisers should not take drugs and medicinal herbs at the same time.

76. To guide qi into your body without draining it, you must strictly follow the methods outlined later. Then you must learn to contract the anal sphincter at the right time and in the right way while guiding qi down in the right way. Careless guiding of the qi will result in problems.

77. One of the most difficult things to master is the

degree of focus of the mind. You must learn from experience. Too many disturbing thoughts make it difficult to focus the mind on the dan tian. Too strong a focus may cause a headache and nervousness. You must decide upon the degree of focus for yourself.

Your mind may begin to focus slowly at first, gradually, from light to strong. Continue until you feel comfortable, as if the mind is on the point. In the beginning the mind may focus a little more strongly in order to get used to the meditation. Also the degree may differ each time in order to adjust to new situations and conditions.

78. Do not fear when half your body feels hot and the other half feels cold, when the body feels hot and cold in turns or when one finger becomes hot and the others remain cold. The cause may be improper gestures or not exercising in the correct way but it could be indicative of a health problem. Just correct the gestures or the exercise. Should it happen again drink some hot water before you exercise and move around so as to make your body warm up naturally; then begin meditation.

79. It is normal to occasionally feel some mild itching, sour stomach, pain, cold, hot, or a puffy or swollen feeling while exercising qigong. If any of these sensations become really strong and make you feel restless, then they would be considered problematic. In such cases remain calm. Continue doing qigong, relax and see if the symptoms go away. If not, and your life becomes affected, stop exercising and get some treatment from a qigong master who is really experienced and good.

80. Control overly-violent movements while doing standing meditation. If you tend to move downward vio-

lently, you should hold your arms straight above your head – above the bai hui point – with the middle fingers touching; then rub the palms vigorously. If you move straight upward violently, you should place your two middle fingers touching over the lower stomach, rubbing your hands vigorously on the middle of the bone of your hands. If you are moving left and right, you may rub your two hands in the front of your chest.

81. If you feel suddenly frightened by some noise or something else while meditating, stop at once. Put your palms on both ears and press gently ten times. Or you may drink a cup of hot tea, then wash your face with a hot towel, or soak your hands in hot water for one or two minutes. The best way is to take a hot bath.

Another way to rectify such a problem is to do "double returning qi" back to the lower Dan Tian eight times. (You can fine this method in the Soaring Crane Qigong book if you want.)

Another way is to do the double returning qi into the bai hui. (You can find the point on one of the included charts.) Then, with palms facing upward and fingers crossed, and with your neck and spine centered, relax the shoulders and push the hands upward. Continuing with the spine centered, push your hands up and bend down to bring both hands to the front, and move hands left and right. Repeat this three times. Then stand up, and use both hands to send qi into the lower dan tian, at the same time contracting the bottom.

82. Do not attempt to treat others when you feel you have gained some power if you have no knowledge of Chinese medicine.

83. You may be able to deal with the problems caused by improper exercise even when there is no qigong master available. If you have identified your error, stop exercising. To correct the problems caused, slap yourself from head to toe along the channels and on the points while relaxing the part being slapped. An alternative is to rub the bottom of the feet – the yong quan points – and with the mind guide the qi down to the bottom of the feet 300 times a day. Maintain a happy mood, do some light work, and keep good thoughts in the mind.

84. For sicknesses, there are different short forms qigong designed by qigong masters or doctors for different cases. For example there are the standing forms for arthritic patients; for patients who have severe stomach problems there are reclining styles; for patients with heart disease (not acute) there is a sitting style; for those whose hearts do not function satisfactorily there is a reclining style with the mind on the upper body, and they may advance to a sitting style later as they recover.

For people who have stomach problems: if you are weak you should choose the free lying style; if your digestion is not good or you are constipated, choose the lying style with legs crossed; if you have gas, choose the lying down style with knees bent and with feet flat on the floor.

85. Any kind of the spontaneous movements can only benefit. If you are losing control of the movements, such as you were going to run, change the gesture. If standing, sit down; if sitting, lie down. Mentally guide yourself to slow down and adjust them. Breathing out slowly can calm the movements. Generally if you are guided by a good teacher there should be no such prob-

lems except, of course, for those with mental disease. It is also possible to help patients who are mentally-diseased, but this should be done only under the guidance of experienced teachers.

86. Qigong comes from six families: Taoism, Buddhism, Confucianism, Wushu (what Westerners eventually named "martial arts"), Chinese medicine, and from local people. It is good to know what type of qigong you are learning.

87. No matter what type, it is important to learn directly from a teacher – a teacher of good moral character. Choose a teacher according to your own need and purpose.

88. Only by cultivating your own good moral character can you learn qigong and improve. The elements of good character include honesty, courage, enthusiasm, service, faith, hope and love.

89. The best time to practice qigong is after midnight and before noon as the qi will be easier to adjust.

90. The hour and length of time you exercise should depend upon your health and age. Usually those who are younger can handle more exercise. Follow the proper steps and make progress step by step. Typical exercise is twice a day for 10 to 60 minutes according to your level of conditioning. The best time is one-half hour before and after meals.

91. The best air temperature for exercise is 15 to

25 degrees C. (60 to 75 degrees F.). Too cold an environment will affect the circulation of the blood. Do not exercise in a thick fog or during thunderstorms.

92. Only those who have practiced qigong for a long time can exercise different kinds of qigong at the same time, and one must schedule them well. This is not for beginners.

93. One can exercise qigong while traveling on a bus or a boat but it must be done in a suitable way.

94. While exercising one may listen to music of the right kind, listening to it as if you were not listening. The volume should be low and unobtrusive.

95. Usually women who are menstruating can practice qigong. Some may experience an increase in the amount of flow; some periods may be lengthened or shortened. To avoid problems, reduce the focus on the dan tian and focus instead on good thoughts or shift the focus of the mind to another spot such as the yong quan. One may reduce the length of the exercise or stop entirely during the time of the period. It is not good to have spontaneous movements during this time. There is no need to become nervous; it is all normal. Should it worsen, however, see a physician or an acupuncturist.

96. Do not contract your bottom (anal area) while doing standing meditation. Should there be an escape of gas let it out naturally.

97. It does not matter whether you keep your eyes

open or closed while doing qigong. It depends upon the person and the situation. The objective is to remain calm, peaceful, and relaxed.

98. The qi and the body work together. The key point is to follow the qi's flowing movement, and not guide it when it is moving.

99. Avoiding the wind is as important as avoiding being shot by an arrow. When exercising, all your pores are open. Even a gentle wind can harm the channels. You should stop exercising when there is strong wind. Close the window if it is windy. Even the sound of wind is not good for the exerciser.

100. To avoid problems:

a.) Follow the rules strictly for the type of gong you are practicing

b.) Maintain a correct, relaxed posture, and smile Relax all parts of the body and especially the forehead

c.) Breath naturally, slowly, and softly

d.) Do not seek any particular desire or feeling

e.) Do not be frightened by sudden shocks or sounds; either continue or slowly end the form.

101. Ending the form correctly will bring greater benefits. Some problems can be caused by ending the form incorrectly. After meditation always place your

palms over the lower dan tian for a while. To finish the
standing meditation always lift both arms above the head,
straighten the legs, turn the palms upward and breath
in. Then, with your palms facing downward, push down
slowly and then mind turn palms facing your lower dan
tian and sending the qi into lower dai tian. Do this three
to five times. Then rub the palms together and massage
the face and head.

102. Do not think of dancing when doing standing
meditation. If you should start to dance a little you should
stop it, otherwise you might start to dance wildly and
lose control. This can cause problems.

103. If the mind is too focused or too absent while
doing qigong, it may cause dizziness or nausea. Such sensations may also happen to a physically weak person who
chooses the standing type; or the movement is too much
work for the person or at the particular time too long or
the exercise is in a windy location. To avoid such problems do everything in the correct way as you have been
instructed.

104. While finishing your moving form, you should
also contract your bottom (the anal sphincter muscle)
and relax your shoulders when guiding qi down to the
dan tian. Contract the bottom in order to avoid draining
the energy and to store the energy in the lower dan tian.
Contracting the bottom also treats emissions, hemorrhoids, and prostate problems.

105. A couple should not make love when they exercise qigong, neither should those who are severely sick.

And for beginners, better not before finishing the 100 days exercise.

106. Treat yourself with your own energy, to open your own channels, to kill germs or to stop or to reduce pain.

107. If you experience problems while exercising qigong, first contact your teacher. Problems are usually of two kinds:

a.) you are over-anxious for quick results; your mind works too hard and causes the qi to become stuck, or

b.) you guide the mind in a disorderly fashion, causing the qi to fail to return to the dan tian, thus causing the qi to become scattered.

With the help of your teacher these problems can be solved quickly.

108. Can one solve his own problems caused by doing qigong in the wrong way?

The answer is "maybe". Breathe out "xu-" or "san-" sounds, as long as you can, to release stuck qi.

To treat scattered qi, breathe out "xu-" or "san-" sounds, and visualize your qi spreading into the outer world as wide as you can, and then imagine it returning back into yourself.

109. The yin and yang energies can lose their balance because of incorrect qigong exercising. If the yang is too high, relax the body, calm the mind and do not focus it; gradually there will be a return to normal. If the

yin energy is too strong, one should increase the work and focus of the mind.

110. Repeating some incantation may also help. Some Grand Masters think the incantations not only guide people to calm down more quickly, but also benefit health. The sounds may resonate inside the body and stimulate the qi. Even repeat them quietly and you will benefit.

111. The essence of a type of gong is often passed on individually, directly by the Grand Master. It is difficult to learn only from a book. Also, a master would avoid teaching the wrong person. To teach the essence, the teacher finds the student. Usually the student does not find the teacher. The master knows what kind of person he wants. A saying is, it takes much longer time for a qigong master to find the right student than a student to find the right teacher.

112. Some who only exercise sitting meditation with legs folded (or only practice the hard gong of the stomach) may get a little large tummy, some may not. Those who do both moving forms and meditation will usually get rid of their big tummy. That is because qigong will improve digestion and sleep. If they are not doing the right form or following the steps correctly, their big tummy might not go away.

Someone may wonder "What about Buddha?" In fact, all those big-tummy Buddha statues and pictures were from people with their overactive imaginations.

113. Many skin problems can be treated and cured by doing qigong. According to Chinese medicine, many

skin diseases are caused by the disorders of the inner secretion system. In Gong Zu's article (Chinese Qigong and Science, 8/94), he wrote how he had treated skin problems caused by disorders of the inner secretion system. Besides medical treatment, the patient may do standing meditation and the moving form to improve (wei channel) circulation and stimulate the blood sent to the tissue.

The qigong types to choose are Youyi Quan standing meditation, Dacheng Quan, Kongjin Qigong, and Shao Lin Yizhichen, among others. Later add sitting meditation to nurture the qi inside your body.

114. Can a person do qigong and other physical exercise at the same time? Yes. They are not in conflict. Physical exercise strengthens the muscles, while qigong strengthens the moving of the inner channels and the qi. Meditation does not seem like moving. Yet it is like exercise for the inside of the body. But you should wait until you calm down to start the qigong exercise. The best result is to do qigong last or before going to bed.

115. People who practice qigong will reduce or even cure body odor.

116. Falling asleep while doing lying meditating will retard progress, or even reduce the gong or drain the qi. To avoid it, you may keep the eyes lightly opened; or keep the mind working more or do the standing or sitting meditation instead of the lying type.

117. One person wrote to explain that the lower half of his body had always felt cold, but after exercising

qigong he often awoke during the night feeling too hot. His stomach felt sore and bloated. This was because he originally lacked the yang qi in his lower body; the increase in yang caused the heat. The stomach sensations indicated the qi was working on some stomach problem. It was a good sign and he only needed to let the qi work.

118. There was someone who had exercised qigong for a while, and felt the qi one day. The movement of the qi would not stop, even after he stopped exercising. He felt it day and night. But it was just the qi working itself. If this happens, let it be. Do not force the mind to guide it. But remember, do not end the exercise before you do the ending form to gather qi into dan tian; focus the mind on lower dan tian for a while.

119. If you run or jog in the morning, always walk until relaxed and calm before exercising qigong.

120. Someone asked if he should follow if the qi in the dan tian turned in one direction. It does not matter. The important thing is to keep the mind on the dan tian slightly. The movement of the qi ball in the dan tian should remind you to keep your mind on the dan tian slightly.

121. Someone asked whether the "Magic Sitting Pad" or the "Magic Pagoda" are really helpful in exercising qigong. It is hard to say just from the advertisements. Many commercials are only for making money. Some may be good, some may be fake.

122. When the good qi washes the sick qi down, will the sick qi get stuck somewhere in the body? No. But

do not fall asleep when thinking that the sick qi is washed away. Follow the next step in your exercise.

123. Someone pointed out the sensation of his nose feeling bigger, and his head expanding, as if someone's shadow was in front of him, etc. But when he opened his eyes, nobody was there. The head feeling is a common reaction, because the good qi is rising. If there are no problems in the head, in about ten days that feeling will be gone. But if there is a problem in the head, such as a tumor, the qi will constantly attack the problem. Sometimes the qi will also work through the yu zhen points (lower back of the head). Then there will be obnoxious noise in the ears and the whole back of the head will feel swollen, even the shoulders and neck. These are all normal reactions; leave them alone. If you can't take any more, you should visualize the inner side of the bai hui point (the top of the head) and help the qi to come through. As soon as the qi starts moving, let it move by itself. Do not be after it.

124. Clean yourself and eliminate wastes before doing qigong. If, in the middle of exercise, you must go, then you must go. It is better not to hold it. But always do the ending form first.

125. Someone asked if the qigong can help someone with several diseases. Yes. Qigong is not like doctors who only treat a certain kind of sickness. Qigong adjusts the balance of the whole body. Thus it is not right to think of choosing one type of qigong to treat one kind of disease, and choosing another to treat another kind of sickness. It's good to learn a complete type of gong and

stick to it. The short forms of qigong were designed by doctors specific for certain diseases and are all based on the formal types.

126. Why is it not good to take antibiotics? Because antibiotics block the qi. Also, consider the side effects, especially taken after a long time.

127. Sometimes antibiotics may be necessary to treat some acute case and save a life; they kill germs and viruses. To take them appropriately and reduce the dose according to your health improvement.

Choosing a Teacher

CHAPTER 10

The best way to learn qigong is to have a good teacher. A good qigong teacher is an ordinary person. The Lord Buddha went to beg alms himself. He helped clean and wash his own bowl after eating.

If a person acts like a god, or deifies himself, it only shows he is infatuated with himself. A good teacher is not greedy for fame or money.

Even if the teacher is really knowledgeable and excellent, he may have some weaknesses. You can learn from his knowledge and not absorb his weaknesses. Respect him either way. The resonance between you and your teacher will only benefit you.

If a master is able to treat many people at the same time, the best way to evaluate him is to see how long the treatment results last afterwards. Of course, one must keep exercising to give the results the opportunity to linger and to stabilize the healing.

Visualization of Channels and Acupoints

CHAPTER 11

This chapter is a translation of Zhang Xioyan's article about qi channels (Qi Gong and Science, Vol.1, 1994):

Dr. Zhong Chuan-yuan of the Beijing Xuan Wu Hospital and I have repeated experiments using The Eight Methods of the Turtle Spirit to time acupuncture treatments. The results summarized below lead to a conceptualization of the movement of qi and the channels through which it flows.

1. The channels are liquid in form. When I observe the inner body, the liquid channels are illuminated by qi and this liquid flows slowly between the tissues of the skin, muscles, organs, and tendons, and is without form unless changed by external influences. When the acupuncture needle is inserted and stimulated at an acupoint, the qi is gathered at that point; energy is expended, making the liquid in the channel flow faster, led by a point of light - the qi. The qi pauses briefly at acupoints where it glows like a star and continues flowing. To summarize:

a.) Channels are at different depths (levels) within the tissues of the body.

b.) Channel sizes vary among people according to age, the size of the individual, health and strength. Everyone is different.

c.) Channel size will also change within the individual as the time of day, different spaces and places influence the body in different ways. Strong or weak movement within the channels will reflect the time of day – whether day or night, sun or moon, the stars and the tides. At its working hour (a specific time) a certain channel will open bigger and stronger and the active qi is the qi of that time. When that channel is open the flow is strong.

d.) Channel sizes vary and the same channel may be a different size in different parts of the body. The twelve main channels and the other eight principal channels may be thought of as rivers and their branches as tributaries that form a crisscross grid throughout the body. Places where they intersect are the main acupoints. The rate of movement of qi is influenced by acupuncture.

e.) When I looked within the channels of the inner body, they appeared like light – of different colors in a definite pattern when given external power. For example, in the four arms the channel color is light blue; inside the body where two channels intersect the point may be red, blue, or light yellow; some crossing points may be blue/purple or the inner one blue and the outer one red. These lights appear as threads or strings, flat or round, or as balls. At the bai hui and the shan gen points the lights are purple and rotate like whirlpools.

2. The shapes of the points and their function:

a. The points connected by the crisscross net or grid are like stars twinkling, large and small, strong and weak and are of different shapes. They spread out at different levels and into spaces within the body. Within the nei guan and the wai guan they appear to be of a flat/round shape (laterally compressed) connected to each other in the middle. If the acupuncture needle is inserted deeply into the nei guan, the wai guan point stretches and qi flows in the wai channel. The bai hui, jing ming, da zhui, and zu san li shine most brightly. Other lesser points are not as bright. All acupoints are three dimensional and have space within. Different points feel different as their shapes are different.

b.) All points store some electrical energy.

c.) Both sides of all points are connected with channels.

d.) All points act as pumps and respond to stimulation from needles and massage. The points respond strongly or weakly according to the energy they receive, and then reproduce energy differently. These points or pumps stimulate qi liquid in the channels and cause it to flow among muscles, nerves, organs, and cells, thereby strengthening blood flow, so as to treat diseases and build up health. Acupuncture and massage can be regarded as energy transfers or energy sources.

3. The positions and shapes of the intersections of the eight principal channels when performing acupuncture according to the hour of The Eight Methods of the Turtle Spirit:

a.) All the points of the yin channels (lie que, zhao

hai, gong sun, and nei guan) join at the tian tu at the throat, then continue in parallel down to the zhong yuan to form a plum-sized pool that feels hot and has a rosy color.

   b.) All the points on the yang channel (such as wai guan, lin shi, hou xi, and zhong mai) meet at the tian mu (around the eyes and nose) and this point or intersection has the shape of a fan shining with rosy-purple light and moving to the left circle in front of the dan tian.

   4. The existence of the zhong mai or Middle Channel: When I practiced qigong or from acupuncture I had an awareness of a straight channel from bai hui to hui ying. At first it was small and fine. After practicing qigong the channel became bigger and later became a crystal clear red pipe. Not everyone has the middle channel or can keep it open. The middle channels among ordinary people are like dotted lines. Use of the middle channel has a special purpose that can be learned only by exercise.

True Stories of Qigong and Tao

CHAPTER 12

1. A couple thousand years ago, there was a monk who wanted to attain tao. He read the classic works of Buddhism. He worshipped each word. After eight years, one day, when he was showing respect to the next word, he suddenly stopped – it was the word "shit".

The monk thought, "Why should I worship the word 'shit'?" At that moment he attained tao.

2. A well-known scholar, Su Dong-po, one day thought he had attained tao. So he wrote to his good friend, a well-known monk. The monk wrote him back, "Your tao is like farting."

Su was angry at the monk's response. He took a boat to cross the river immediately; he was ready to argue. But the monk said nothing. Instead, he wrote a poem: "One fart has driven you to cross the river." Su then realized that he was far from attaining tao.

3. Something happened in Vietnam when the Chinese soldiers were sent there to help build the hidden cannon front. It was in June, 1965, in the suburb of Beining City, Hepei province. The Chinese troops had just finished building the front.

After lunch a group of five soldiers hung out and walked around the hill. Then they went into one of one of the hideouts. These young men wanted to see how the thick, rubber-covered door worked. It was for protection from chemical weapons. But after they closed the door, there was no way for them to reopen it, no matter what they had tried. They were completely stuck in the dark cave because nobody could hear them.

Eventually they became worn out by trying to open it, and became worried. One of the five soldiers had learned qigong from his grandfather when he was little. He suggested that in order to survive and wait for the rescue, they had to learn qigong from him. His grandfather had told him that when there was no food, qigong could help save his life. So they had to learn from the young man. They lay on the ground, learned and exercised it all the time, and only stopped when they went to urinate or drink water. They had no idea how long they had been inside the cave, until one day, the door was suddenly opened and they were saved. They had been in there fourteen days! They were sent to the hospital, and all were fine. After that, the other four soldiers were qigong lovers.

4. Genghis Khan, the Mongolian emperor and infamous invader, practiced qigong. Before he started his invasions, he consulted a well-known Taoist, Qiu Chu-ji, and learned qigong from him. Even now, in Inner Mongolia, the historical record of his life story and about how he had learned qigong from the Taoist is still kept. Unfortunately he killed many people, which was not a Taoist ideal.

5. The first Chinese emperor, Shen Nong, according to history, was also a Grand Qigong Master. He had all the super powers as Jesus, and as that the contemporary Grand Masters have. He could see through the human body, and see which herbs went to which channels and organs. He taught people the nature of herbs and

how to use them to treat diseases.

History records much about Lao Tzu, Lord Buddha, and Jesus, and showed that all these sages were able to treat people's diseases, were able to see through people's bodies, were able to walk on the surface of water, etc.

6. A Chinese emperor (about 907-960) once asked the Fourth Buddhist originator, "I have built so many temples and donated so much money, how am I doing? Have I done enough good deeds to become a Buddha?"

The monk answered, "You have done none."

7. When Dr. Nan Hui-jin was young, the wife of a friend wanted to become a student of a Buddhist scholar - Dr. Nan's teacher. But the old man refused her.

She felt wronged, and swore she would teach herself by reading books. She did sitting meditation for a long time. One day, while sleeping, she dreamed that the Buddha invited her to heaven, and she enjoyed many things. Then she thanked Buddha and went home because she was worried about her husband.

Suddenly a female ghost appeared in front of her. The woman was not afraid and said to the ghost, "You look so ugly, I would be ashamed to show up before people if I were you!" The ghost felt embarrassed and was gone.

After a while, a handsome man showed up, but she knew that it was just the female ghost – who had changed into a man. She told the man what she thought and told him to go away. Instead, the man changed into such a ferocious ghost that she was terrified. She ran and ran for all she was worth, until, at her home gate she fell down exhausted.

She then woke up, and realized it was a dream. She

sat up, thinking and thinking. She awoke her husband and told him about her dream. In telling it, she began to understand. "Now I see," she said. "The Buddha was me, and the female ghost was me, and both the man and the terrifying ghost were me, too! They all came from my mind."

The next day she went to visit that old scholar. Before she could begin to tell him her dream, he smiled and said, "I know everything. Now you may become my student."

Short-Form Self-Healing Gong

CHAPTER 13

The present growing interest has encouraged me to translate some forms what I call the Short-Forms of qigong. These are more properly called the Short-Forms because most of them have been cultivated by qualified people who have exercised qigong for years. These forms are based on their experience and knowledge. Some of them are chosen by the masters from a formal type. The short forms usually only have one form, unlike the formal types designed by the Grand Masters or handed down from ancient times, although these Short-Forms are based upon them. Formal types are a special subset of qigong forms, they are practiced by starting with a beginning level, and moving on through progressively more advanced levels. Many of them are taught by the Grand Masters themselves only, and have been passed on for many generations.

These Short-Forms are designed to treat different problems. They can help qigong lovers, and also help those who can't afford expensive doctors and want to avoid harmful drugs. Different individuals have different needs, like different plants need different environments. Some need plenty of sunlight, some need shade, some need more water, some need well-drained soil. Different people have different degrees of ability to absorb and send qi. But everyone is able to develop this ability, if he or she does qigong continuously. The following will give you some guidelines as you learn qigong.

Though the different types of qigong differ, they all address the same overall goal: to improve health, and to approach much more than that. You choose the kind that you feel comfortable with. These short forms of qigong are *only* for people who have practiced qigong regularly for at least three months and have some knowledge of qigong.

To start learning qigong, the best way is to consult a qigong teacher, and to choose the right kind for you. In order to learn and improve, you must retain a peaceful, relaxed mind, be kind to others, and do good deeds. Then you'll learn qigong well. When you feel badly about yourself because you have done something bad, you will feel guilty, and the guilty feeling will remain in your subconscious. Negative feelings like this can disturb your qi.

But when you decide to change, the good feelings will help your qi circulate better and improve your qigong. Some Grand Qigong Masters request their students to serve the society and do good deeds. People's praise and love will return positive energy. This will benefit the students as they practice qigong.

Remember the most important rules when you exercise qigong:

1. The tip of your tongue lightly touches the maxilla (in some special methods it may be positioned differently).

2. You must understand the real meaning of some of the requests while doing qigong. "To close your eyes", for example, means to keep the outside world outside, and to retain a calm, peaceful mind, and forget how you feel. If you can't be in such a state, simply closing your eyes will not help, although you have to learn to do it gradually. "To relax" does not mean only the body and the mind, but also any tense part of your body.

3. Follow the steps strictly. Each movement is designed for a reason. It is not only the physical exercise. Most importantly, you must follow the steps for the movement of qi along the channels. You will understand the reasons after you exercise for a while. It may be a long time until you learn to feel the qi moving.

4. If one type of qigong does not work for you, maybe there is something wrong with the way you are exercising. It may be the time or the place. If you choose to consider a different type of qigong, do not change frequently – it won't do you good. Each individual is different, and is sensitive to different things. Finally, different people will progress differently.

5. When some part of your body feels more sensitive about qi than the other parts, you should pay more attention to it; you'll improve more quickly.

1. HEEL LIFT

Feet, which carry the body's weight, are the body part furthest away from the heart. A foot contains thousands of nerve endings, 26 bones, 33 joints, 50 ligaments, 50,000 blood vessels and over 40,000 sweat glands. Repeatedly lifting the heels off the ground will stimulate the movement of nerve endings, glands, and ligaments, and help the blood vessels function better so as to accelerate blood circulation and improve the immune system.

Also, according to Chinese medicine theory, there are a total of 12 channels that start in the feet (zu san yang channel, zu san yin channel). These 12 channels contain 422 acupoints. Lifting the heels in coordination with inhalation and exhalation pushes, pulls, presses, massages, and directly works the acupoints on the 12 channels, so as to prevent and treat diseases.

According to the ancient Chinese Foot Massage book, the bottom of each foot has 35 reactive areas. On the outer ankle there are 22 reactive areas while the inner ankle has 16. Each foot has a total of 73 reactive points. Briefly, all organs and all parts of the body have a corresponding reactive area in the foot.

The exercise:

Lift your heels while inhaling as slowly and deeply as you can, then return your heels slowly to the ground while exhaling.

There has been observational research on a group of 20 people, male and female, all over the age of 58 who practice this gong. The participants have been exercising this gong for one to two years. All 20 people showed improvement in their health: seven who had heart diseases at the onset of this research have almost completely recovered; four diabetic patients have completely recovered; one woman's breast tumor is gone and none of these people have had any brain diseases develop.

2. INTELLIGENCE-DEVELOPING QIGONG
By Grand Master Yan Xin

Preparation: Sit in a chair that will allow your knees to be bent at a 90-degree angle to the floor, knees against each other tightly and feet together making full contact with the ground. Sit near the front of the chair keeping your back straight and not touching the back of the chair. Relax your chest and shoulders, do not keep them rigid. Keep your head straight upward and lower your chin slightly. Relax. Eyes may be either open or closed. The exercise contains five steps.

The exercise:

a.) Place your left palm 2.5 inches away from the zhong ji (five inches below the navel).

b.) Place your right palm on the left side of the chest, 2.5 inches away from the nipple. Keep the shoulders, elbows, wrists and fingers relaxed. Breath naturally for a while.

c.) Begin to count the breaths. At first, only count the inhale, 120 times; then count the exhale only, also 120 times.

d.) While counting the inhales, imagine many hot light rays being absorbed in from the hui yin (the point between the anus and genitals). During the exhalation imagine the qi being breathed out from the yu zhen (the two points down the occipital bones). Both the inhalation and exhalation should be as slow, soft, and even as possible.

e.) During the whole exercise, think of your right palm sending light to lighten your heart.

f.) After the inhaling and exhaling exercise, slowly lift your left hand up to the top of your head, approximately 2.5 inches from your head, palm facing downward. Circle counterclockwise above your head beginning from the back, to the right, to the front, etc. Move slowly imagining that the qi is being absorbed through the bai hui (the point on top of the head in the middle between your two ears). The number of circles depends on a person's health: a healthy person may circle 49 times, a weak person should circle seven times.

Completion: When finished with the circling, move your left hand slowly down from the front of your body to 2.5 inches in front of the tummy, and visualize the qi going down from the top of your head to your lower dan tian. Move your right hand down at the same time. Keep the right hand on the left hand and the thumbs crossed. Think of the qi gathering into the dan tian.

To get best results, do this exercise between 11:00 p.m. and 1:00 a.m., and on holidays. The energy that groups bring together is much more powerful than individual energy. The more people that exercise together - the more they will benefit each other.

3. SELF-TREATING STOMACH PAIN
By Lin Shiming and Li Hanqin

From many years of our own practice and experience, we have summarized this short-form gong for treating stomach pain caused by: being weak and afraid of the cold (when pressing the lower stomach the person feels pain or fullness of fluids); and feeling stuffy, with no appetite (when pressing the stomach the person will feel pain, or suffer from constipation). This is not for acute cases.

Self treatment steps:

a.) Wear casual, comfortable clothes. Either sit, cross legged, or lie on your back. Place both hands on your navel; males place the right hand on top of the left hand, women to the contrary. Relax, close your eyes slightly, and breath naturally. When inhaling, think of heat flowing from your esophagus into your belly. In the beginning, the breathing may be irregular but in a few minutes it will become smooth and you will feel better and your stomach will gradually become warm. End the gong when you feel physically good.

b.) Then, if the pain is caused by cold, you should move your hand clockwise on the belly 30 times. If the pain is caused by feeling too full, stuffiness, you should move your hands counterclockwise 30 times.

4. SELF TREATING SLEEPLESSNESS

When you cannot sleep, try to keep these thoughts constantly in your mind, quietly: the sky is high...I am as high as the sky...the earth is big...I am as large as the earth...I am standing on a piece of wooden board, the blue sky is under my feet...the space is boundless and full of qi...my qigong teacher is with me....

After repeating this a few times, you will fall asleep soundly. After a time, your sleep disorder will be cured.

5. SELF TREATING LOWER BACK PAIN

Lower back pain, caused by the kidneys being weak, can be treated with this gong. The posture can be sitting, lying, or standing, in whatever way you feel comfortable. Use your mind to imagine that your eyes are looking at your two kidneys for a minute. Beginners may start using their hands to send qi into their kidneys. At the same time, imagine the ming men (the middle point between the kidneys on the spine) and shen yu (at the two kidney spots) are open, and all the good qi from the universe is streaming into the kidneys. In a while, your kidney spots will feel warm.

Finish with the ending form: use your mind to imagine lifting your kidneys up nine times, then pat the kidney spots with palms, not fully touching them. Exercise one or two times a day; the duration and time of day are up to you.

After you have exercised for many days and mastered the method, you can stop using your hands to send qi. Just imagine two big, invisible hands are sending qi into your kidneys and ming men.

This method benefits the kidney yang energy and builds up the kidney's yin energy. After exercising for a long time, you won't catch cold easily, nor be afraid of cold.

6. SELF TREATING CERVICAL VERTEBRAE PROBLEMS

Preparation for the exercise: stand with your feet as wide as your shoulders and relax, with your eyes looking forward, seeing nothing:

a.) Lower your head as low as you can, trying to reach your chest. Then slowly straighten your head to an upright position. Move your head back as far as you can, then return to an upright position again slowly. Lean your head to the left side as low as you can and then return to the center. Move your head to the right side as far as you can and then return to an upright position in the center.

b.) Turn your head slowly to the left, then slowly from the left to the back as far as you can. Your eyes should look at the ground to the left, and then behind you on the ground. Repeat this sequence on the right side, performing the moves to the right respectively.

c.) Turn your head slowly to the left, then to the back. This time as you turn your head look up to the sky in each direction your head turns. Return to the original position. Repeat this sequence to the right.

d.) With your head, neck and shoulders relaxed, roll your head from left, to back, to right, to front (counterclockwise) nine times. Repeat this clockwise nine times.

e.) Stand in the preparation posture and make your hands into fists hanging at your waist, pushing the muscles on both sides of the spine toward the spine as tightly as possible. Your elbows will come toward your body as you push. At the same time, push your head and neck forward as far as you can, sticking out your chin, eyes forward. Return to the preparation position, relax. Repeat this a few times.

f.) Stand in the preparation posture this time with fingers crossed in front of your belly, palms facing up. Lift your palms up to the chest, then flip your hands over so that when you raise your hands palm up above your head your thumbs are facing forward. Lean your head back and look at your little fingers.

Separate your hands and bring them down to your sides at shoulder level, palms facing backwards and up, with thumbs apart from the other fingers. Focus your eyes on the left four fingers. Move back to the preparation posture. Repeat this four times. Then do the same on the right side.

g.) From the standing posture again, the right hand reaches up and over the right shoulder down the back; the left hand reaches down and around the left side to meet the fingers of the right hand and hold them (if it is too difficult to hold the fingers just make sure they are facing each other). Turn waist, shoulders, neck, and head to the left-back, as far as you can with eyes looking back. Then slowly come back to center, standing posture. Repeat this one to four times. Repeat this entire sequence on the right side.

h.) In the standing posture, rub the palms together until they are hot. Then use the right hand to massage the upper front of the left shoulder (the points: jian jing, tian mu, qu hen, bing feng, tian zong, ru yu, ju gu, jian niu) and down the arm. Then use the left palm to massage the right side in the same manner. Repeat three times. Now use the right palm to massage from the upper back (da zhui point to jing bai lao, tian zhu, jian zhong yu, jian wai yu, jian jing) to the shoulder. Use the left palm to massage the right side in the same sequence. (If this is difficult to do by yourself, ask someone to help). Do this two to three times a day.

7. BABY QIGONG
By kindergarten teacher Tsai Baozhen, (2/95)

When telling a short story, tell the children (three years old or younger) to sit with legs crossed, thumb and middle fingers touching, and hands on knees. Then, let each baby hold a ball, and tell them to imagine they are sitting in a rocking chair on flowing water. Then tell them to look into the water. Or, tell them they are flying in a space ship and seeing many wonderful scenes. Play for a while, then do the ending form: simply cross their hands on their tummies and listen to another short story.

A month after doing this the change in my children was obvious. Through two years of experimentation all my children have done better in all other classes. They are healthier and more intelligent, and their ability to handle things has improved. I have also written a qigong dance for little children.

8. WALKING QIGONG

Walking gong has been prescribed by Chinese doctors for treating chronic and complicated cases.

Preparation: sit naturally and straight; imagine there is a gold circle on your navel. Do this for one to fifteen minutes depending on your condition. Then you may begin your walk.

Walk one to two times a day, for half an hour each time. Walk evenly, steadily, body relaxed, without thinking, mind peaceful and calm. Do not use a personal radio. Do not talk or stop. A weak person may adjust the speed so that they don't become overtired.

Ending form: sit quietly for one to fifteen minutes.

9. HOW I CURED MY SHOULDER
By Zhang Dongsheng (11/94)

When I was six years old I fell off a tree and injured my left shoulder. Since then, I have always had a twitch in my left shoulder and felt as if there was something in it, very uncomfortable. After practicing qigong for several years, I started thinking about treating my shoulder. I imagined there was a sun inside my left shoulder, flames spreading, melting the coldness and uncomfortable feeling inside. Then the feelings left when the flames went out. It took me ten minutes to finish this exercise. After a few times my shoulder was amazingly cured!

10. SELF TREATING COLD

There are two methods for treating cold, and either may be used.

Method A: Sit straight in a chair, chin lowered slightly, tongue touching your maxilla. Place both palms on your knees, eyes lightly closed. Keep your mind focused on the lower dan tian, relaxed. After a while bring your arms up to the front shoulder level and bring your hands to the front of your nose and send qi toward your nose 30 times. Now place your left hand on top of your right hand (males place right on left) and bring them approximately 2.5 inches away from your nose. Move them counterclockwise 15 times. Now hold your breath and keep your mind focused on the nose point. Breathe deeply, inhaling and exhaling six to nine times. Move your hands back to your knees again and rest for a while. Repeat this entire sequence a few times.

Method B: Sit as in Method A. Lift the buttocks and keep your mind on the lower dan tian. Relax for two to three minutes. Imagine the qi from the dan tian going down to the buttocks and then up the spine to the top of the head, down to the nose and the qi then turning counterclockwise in the nose 30 times and then clockwise 30 times. Focus on the inner side of the nose for about five minutes imagining that you are inhaling and exhaling through all the points on the nose. Now breathe deeply for approximately five minutes. Rest for a while. This exercise takes 10-12 minutes.

11. YIN YANG DA HUA GONG

This gong helps you achieve the meditational state and establish the ability to maintain higher gong.

Quietly sit for a while (in whatever posture you prefer) and imagine you are traveling in the woods, mountains, and parks, all the time leaving your body where it is sitting. Then imagine that winter is gone and spring has arrived with flowers in full blossom. You are on a tour, visiting well-known beautiful places; you can feel the stars in the sky. After a while, you return to the place where your body is sitting, doing qigong.

12. STRENGTHENING THE INNER ORGANS

a.) For the kidneys:

From a standing position, lift both arms up slowly, palms facing each other, to above the head imagining you are holding a big ball of qi from the space around you. Gently rock your head, waist, and stomach allowing the arms to move but not the hands. Then slowly bring down your arms along your side and then move your hands to the lower dan tian, move along the waist with hands moving slowly backward to the kidney spots (make sure not to touch your clothes). At the same time tighten your buttocks including your tailbone so as not to lose qi. Simultaneously swallow the saliva imagining that you are sending it down to the ming men and the kidneys three to seven times. Now cover the kidneys with your hands and think, "Mei shi le (everything is fine now)."

b.) For the heart:

Stretch both arms back from the sides of your hips with your hands gesturing as if you are grasping something. Imagine that your hands are absorbing clear, sweet spring water from streams deep under the ground. Then bring the "water" back up to wash your eyes, then the bai hui (the top of your head), the your heart. Repeat this exercise until you feel cool and good, then stop and sit quietly or stand for awhile.

c.) For the liver:

Lift both hands up above the head (thinking of lifting qi with them) and move the fingers as if playing a piano for about ten seconds. Slowly bring the hands down to the liver thinking that your liver is expanding, becoming endless, and your body changes into the blue sky. Then rest quietly for a while.

d.) For the lungs:
Hold your thumbs with the index and middle finger of each hand. Stretch your hands behind you from under your armpits and arch your back while leaning your head backwards also. Your hands should be facing each other at a 90-degree angle. Breathe out through your nose making the sound "heng-". Repeat eight times.

e.) For the spleen:
Use both palms to gently "massage" the liver and spleen without touching your clothes. Do this gently as if you are massaging two thin-shelled eggs, for about one to two minutes. After you feel good, stop massaging and quietly enjoy the good feeling for a while. Then place both hands down at your sides and relax with eyes closed for a while.

13. FOR PREVENTING PROBLEMS WHILE EXERCISING QIGONG

This gong helps strengthen the mind. Keep doing it and you will become gentle and huge hearted.

Lift both arms from the sides up to ear level, palms down, index fingers pointing away from the body. Imagine that your fingers are pointing out into space. Then quickly imagine that the fingers absorb qi back (like a rubber band snapping back). Bring the index fingers to the middle of the ears, 2.5 inches away, and draw circles in your ears with your index fingers without moving your hands until the fingers feel warm. Bring your hands down to your sides, eyes closed, and imagine that within your body the spring sun is sending rays and warming up your body. Do this for a few minutes.

14. INTELLIGENCE DEVELOPMENT

Place both palms on the sides of the forehead at the temples with fingers pointing toward the center of your forehead. Close your eyes in a meditative state for a while. Move hands upward rubbing against your head. Repeat this a few times, then think calmly.

Another gong for developing intelligence is to use the palms to tap the forehead and then tap the temples for one to two minutes. Then use your five fingers to comb your hair starting at the forehead and moving over and down the back of your head. No prescribed time or time limits. Allow the mind to feel the affects of being combed by the fingers. For and ending form bring your hands down to the dan tian for a minute.

15. FOR NEARSIGHTEDNESS

Close your eyes and imagine that the stars, the moon, and the sun are all covering your body with light, until you feel warm. Inhale and exhale 108 times. Then imagine that your feet are "listening" to water waves deep down under the ground. Inhale and exhale another 108 times. Now open your eyes and look at people, trees, white clouds in the blue sky or mountains. Inhale and exhale another 108 times.

It takes approximately 108 days to heal your eyes.

16. QIGONG FOR STUDENTS
By high school teacher Li Yunxia

I've taught in school for many years and practiced qigong for over ten years. Two minutes before class starts, I ask my students to sit in meditation, one palm on another facing upward but not touching. Their eyes are closed or looking at the tips of their noses. Feet are together with the bottom touching the floor, relaxed. I ask them to keep all monkey-minded thoughts down in the lower stomach, then think of nothing, yet imagine standing in a vast field, or on the beach, or floating in the blue sky for a minute. Now imagine that a very bright sun is rising from the lower stomach, lighting the whole body, lighting the course material they learned last time and also the chapter the teacher is about to teach. After two minutes, they finish the gong and the class begins.

I also often teach them qigong after school. My many years of experimenting with teaching students qigong two minutes before class has helped all my classes do better academically. They also are more healthy than other classes.

17. SLEEPING GONG

If your pillow is too high, it may cause cervical vertebrae problems. If it is too low, it will affect the qi to flow backward, which is not good for the brain. Many people put their pillows even under their shoulders, which should not be done. It should be under the occipital bone where the two yu zhen points are. In this way, the body fluids flow best to the brain. When you lie on a pillow, if your eyes can see the yong quan (arch and instep of your foot) then the height of your pillow is correct. Then the qi will flow automatically in the right direction and you will be maintaining the qigong state while sleeping...the qigong continues. (The above is not for patients who need clinical care.)

18. SCRATCHES AND SCRAPES

A healthy old couple in their late seventies shared their secrets with me: they each spend about ten minutes scratching and scraping the other's back before sleeping. They use fingernails or something else and slightly scratch and scrape repeatedly starting from the neck, down the shoulders then to the middle of the back, the waist, hips, and arms. Along the spine is the most important part. When the person feels hot, they then switch.

19. CONDITIONAL BREATHING WAY

There are many seasons each with their own temperature and humidity level. Therefore, there is a breathing gong that will be good for the health in each season. Doing this gong often, during the appropriate season, will benefit your health. When the weather is dry, you should exhale using the sound "hu-", and take more naps. When it is damp, exhale using the sound "tsuo-" and be more active. When it is hot and humid use the sound "xu-" when exhaling. All these sounds are made with a slow, soft inhale followed by a long exhale.

20. FOR ANAL HEMORRHOIDS

Step A (Standing preparation): Move the feet apart, slightly wider than your shoulders, and bend the knees a little, with both hands in front of the navel as if holding a ball. Close your eyes and imagine there is a small red ball 1.5 inches below the navel. Let your mind guide the ball down. Move the ball down through the outer sexual organs and up to the tail bone to the back ming men point (the point on the lower back opposite the navel) and then return to the navel. Repeat until this route feels smooth.

Step B. Straighten the body. Move your right foot next to your left foot. Keep your hands naturally at your sides. Lift the heels up off the ground and form your hands into tight fists. At the same time inhale and lift the hui yin (middle point between anus and genitals). Hold this posture for a minute. Let the heels come back to the ground suddenly, sharply, while letting go of the fists. Exhale and loosen the hui yin. Repeat nine times.

Step C (Ending form): Rub the hands together until hot. Place them on the stomach near the navel. Females place the left hand on top of the right hand, males do the opposite. Massage in a counter-clockwise direction first for nine circles, then clockwise nine circles. At the same time, with good intention, gather good qi into the dan tian, clearing all the channels and making the hemorrhoids disappear.

(This gong is not for patients who keep bleeding or have severe pain.)

21. SIX CHANT INCANTATIONS
By Pang Tsaixing (9/94) and Zhaorige Tu

The six sounds are from Tibetan Buddhism - Mizong. I was lucky to have learned them from my master Liu Zhao-lin. Once I wanted to treat a black mole under my left lower eyelid – it was considered a bad omen. When I was chanting the six sounds, I purposely chanted loudly, thinking to "shoot away" the mole into the sky. One day in the autumn of 1992, I suddenly found the mole had disappeared! However, I don't remember the exact date when it disappeared. I also know someone whose cancer of the esophagus was cured three months after my master had taught her to chant.

The six sounds are: wong-m, ma ni, bei mei, hong.

Steps (you can also chant quietly in sitting meditation posture): Before starting, smile with your eyes closed. Relax, smile, think of sweet dew water going into the bai hui (top of your head) and wash all over your body with this water. Let it drain from the bottom of your feet. Do this three times. Then chant for about ten minutes, then quietly meditate, thinking of nothing. Or, you can simply do the chanting for a longer period until you feel well.

The meaning of the six sounds:

1) wong-m means to trust and respect Guanyin (a Buddha, often appearing as a female) and the Grand Master. This sound vibrates the whole head and the five areas (eyes, nose, mouth, tongue, and ears). While chanting, think of all the sickness disappearing and you feeling better.

2 & 3) ma, ni means things turn out as you wish and are wonderful. These sounds vibrate the throat area. While chanting, think of all disease in the larynx disappearing and becoming well.

4 & 5) bei mei means there is a beautiful lotus flower in your heart. It grows out of mud; straight, clean and strong. These sounds vibrate the chest. Imagine they are sweeping out all depressed feelings and you feel relaxed and happy.

6) hong means the qigong is functioning effectively. This sound vibrates the lower stomach and funnels the qi into the lower dan tian.

You may start slowly, memorizing the chanting sounds first. Then you divide your body into four chanting vibrational areas: head, throat, chest, and lower stomach. After you can feel the qi, try to feel how the qi follows the sounds, and how it goes through the ren channel (the middle line on your chest). After you have learned them, chant the six sounds continuously.

After you have become familiar with the sounds and

master them, you may try to choose sounds that will clear blockages in your channels.

One time, I divided my chanting areas into six, starting from the bai hui down to the yong quan (top of the head to the bottom of the feet). I divided my body into six vibrational areas: the lower dan tian, the hui yin, the jia bei, the yu zhen (bottom of occipital bone), and the upper dan tian (forehead area). I formed these areas into one line while chanting. Sometimes when I didn't feel too well, I would chant "hong-" and at the end of the chanting I would focus on the ends of my fingernails and toenails imagining that the sick qi was leaving through them.

Later, after I mastered the sounds and experienced strong qi I was able to control the flow of energy, guiding the sound anywhere I wished. For example, I can guide the qi into the air, or to bring back a message from my master when I am chanting the sound "wong-m" and the sound reaches the sky. "Ma-, ni-" vibrates my bai hui and surges into my upper dan tian." Bei mei-" vibrates my middle dan tian. And chanting "hong-" directly sends the energy into my lower dan tian.

Also, there is no time factor for this chanting; no limitation of site or concern of conflicting effects from other types of qigong.

Some other hints: When you exhale more through the left side of your nose than the right, you are in the best state of exercising qigong.

Ending form: Lightly tap your head with an open hand, then guide the qi down with your hands to the lower dan tian.

Alternate ending form: hold your hands together without palms touching, above your head. Then bring your hands down, fingers facing each other, slowly down to the lower dan tian. Imagine that the qi goes down into the lower dan tian.

Cross your fingers in front of the lower dan tian with palms facing the body. Keep your mind on the lower dan tian for about three minutes, imagining the energy from the universe streaming into your Dan Tian continuously.

Then, with your hands on the back of your neck, move them to along the back of your ears, massage up to the top of your head, down to your eyes and massage your eyes for a minute. Then move them up to the head again and down to the back of your neck. Repeat this nine times. Slowly open your eyes and gently massage your legs and the bottom of your feet.

22. PAN GU GONG FOR TREATING
SCAPULOHUMERAL PERIARTHRITIS

After the first ten days of exercising, your shoulder will feel more painful; this shows the qi is treating your shoulders. Don't stop but continue with the exercising. After another ten days, the pain will decrease drastically. In another ten days your shoulder will be healed.

Step A: From a standing meditation posture, inhale and exhale through the nose, thinking that you are as high as the sun. When you are inhaling you are rising and countless sun lights are lighting through the back of your hands, to your palms, along the inner side of your arms, to your shoulders, head, shan zhong (middle of the nipples) and down to the dan tian. Now exhale with no mental work, just naturally and relaxed. Exercise for

30 minutes.

Step B: Hold both arms straight forward, palms facing upward at a 75-degree angle from the ground, wrists slightly bent with fingers pointing upward. When inhaling, pull back the upper arms with palms and fingers tilted slightly; imagine the qi going into the palms along the inner sides of your arms to your shoulders and head, then to the shan zhong, and down to the dan tian. Then exhale naturally without mental work, and bring your arms back to your sides, relaxing your arms and wrists. Repeat this 49 times.

Step C: Hold the arms up, parallel to your sides, palms downward. Inhale and pull the forearms toward your body without moving the upper parts. Keep the fingers facing up and the palms facing the body. The upper arms and lower arms form a 90-degree angle. Imagine the qi coming through the palms and along the inner side of the arms to the shoulders, head, and shan zhong, then down to the dan tian. Exhale without any mental work and bring your arms down to your sides. Repeat this 49 times.

Ending form: Cross both arms over the chest. Reach to your shoulders and rub both shoulders simultaneously, 49 times.

23. FOR DYSFUNCTIONAL SEX ABILITY

Any posture is fine. Allow your eyes to "look" inside your body. Inhale and hold the bottom (male: penis and testicles; female: vagina to anus) then deep into the lower stomach. Exhale and relax all the parts being held including the lower stomach. Do this 18-36 times, twice a day.

From a sitting meditation posture with legs crossed, breathe naturally with the eyes closed. Keep the mind on the qi hai, then the guan yaun, then the hui yin, allowing your eyes to follow internally. Repeat this over and over without a time limit. Do this several times a day.

These two exercises may be done one after another. However, you must do them every day to see an effect.

24. FOR TREATING GUM PROBLEMS
By Wang Shoulu (1/94)

With your mouth closed use your tongue to massage the outside of your gums 36 times. Do not swallow your saliva; allow it to rinse the inside of your mouth as you massage the gums. Then divide the saliva into three portions and slowly swallow each, sending it into the lower dan tian. Do this several times a day. You may also do this while jogging or any activity. I cured myself after doing this for two months.

25. FOR HIGH BLOOD PRESSURE

Frequently focus your mind on the yong quan (bottom of the feet) and exhale slowly, evenly, and as softly as possible. Move your lower body often, as in walking.

26. FOR CATARACTS

First, think a good thought, and think of it when you are exercising, such as: "My eyes are well and bright." Send the message down into the eyeballs.

When doing this exercise, think: "San, tong, lian (the opaque quality in your eyes has disappeared, all your channels are open and clear, your eyes are bright and well)." The more times you say it, the better.

The exercise:

Step A (Sitting or standing meditation posture): relax, eyes open, thinking of absorbing qi into your eyes. Look upward, inhale; exhale and look downward. Do this six times. Then close your eyes and rest. Repeat six times.

Step B: With eyes open, think of qi coming into your eyes, then inhale and look left; exhale and look right. Do this six times, then close your eyes and rest. Repeat six times.

Step C: Open your eyes and gather qi, inhale with your eyes looking upward and to the left; exhale looking downward and to the right. Do this six times. Close your eyes and rest. Repeat six times.

Step D: With eyes open and absorbing qi, inhale and look up and to the right; exhale and look down and to the left. Do this six times. Close your eyes and rest. Repeat six times.

Step E: With eyes open and gathering qi, rotate your

eyes counter clockwise, then clockwise. As your eyes move from down to up inhale; as you move from up to down exhale. Do this six times. Close your eyes and rest. Repeat six times.

Step F: Close your eyes tightly, inhale and exhale slowly, softly, and evenly three times. Then open your eyes wide and look as far as you can. It is best to look at something green. Inhale and exhale three more times, then look at the tip of your nose. Inhale and exhale the same way three times. Repeat the above six times.

Step G: With eyes closed, rub your hands together until they become very hot. Then place the palms over the eyes (with eyes open) and breath naturally six times. Blink eyes eight times. Repeat the above three times.

Ending form: take your hands away from your eyes and bring them down to your navel. At the same time swallow saliva in three portions. Each time you swallow inhale and imagine the saliva going down to the liver to wash it, then to the kidneys and down to the navel. Repeat this three times, two or three times a day.

27. EXERCISING THE CHANNELS: LYING AND BREATHING

This is an important way of exercising your channels. Lie on your back, relax, and breath naturally; keep the mind on the lower dan tian. Do not move your body or chest; inhale slowly, softly, and deeply down into the dan tian. Loosen the stomach muscle and fill it with qi as much as possible until the lower stomach rises up to its maximum height. Hold this for a while. Then exhale and let out as much air as possible until the lower stomach reaches its minimum height. Inhale and exhale the whole time naturally. Exercise two times a day for five to fifteen minutes. Sometimes you may fall asleep while doing it. That is okay. However, do not do this immediately after eating.

This exercise can also be done in the sitting posture.

28. THE SLEEPING WAY OF A SUPERNATURAL BEING

There are four steps:

a.) Males and females do this similarly. In the sitting meditation posture, hold the thumbs, middle, and small fingers of the opposite hands touching as if a ball is held between the hands in front of your lower stomach. Inhale and exhale slowly, deeply, 24 times.

b.) Before lying down to sleep, think of the goodness and wonders of doing qigong, and the master's expression, to enter the qi state.

c.) Males lie on your right side with your right palm on your right ear hole. Keep the right leg nearly straight out and the left leg curled up on the right leg, left hand on the left hip, palm on the huan tiao point, or on the lower stomach. Females do this lying on the left side.

d.) In the morning, before getting up, do the ending

form first: both hands gathering qi into dan tian two or three times.

29. SUPERNATURAL WAYS OF SITTING

Straighten the body and head, moving both arms like boat oars. Bai hui (the top of the head) is gathering the sun, the moon, and the stars into your body; your yong quan (bottom of feet) is gathering water, fire, and wind. All your pores are open and absorbing the good qi from the natural world.

30. SUPERNATURAL SITTING

Imagine that you are sitting in a beautiful lotus flower. A string goes from your head at the bai hui, up to the heavens. Qi is lifting your bottom, and you are surrounded by qi, inside and out.

31. FOR AGED PEOPLE
(THREE-ONE-TWO EXERCISE)

The "three," three points:

a.) He Gu (the point is at the joint part between thumb and index finger),

b.) Zu Zan Li (four fingers down the kneecap. It takes care of digestion, blood presure, joints pain and many other problems), and c.) Nei Guan (the middle point three fingers away from the bottom on the wrist joint.)

Massage the three points twice a day, five minutes each time. The best result is gained when massaging, you feel hot pins or a cold sensation (one minute might mean massaging 30 times).

The "one" - a breathing exercise. Deeply and slowly inhale and exhale down to the lower stomach, twice a day, five minutes each time.

The "two" - two legs. Walking or moving around, five minutes each time, once a day.

The total exercise requires only 25 minutes a day. It helps elderly people stimulate and excite the circulation of their channels.

Tips: The he gu point is on the channel along the outer arm, all the way up to the nose. To massage it frequently and for a long time will prevent or treat facial disease. The nei guan is on the channel up to the lungs and heart (along the inner side of the arm channel) and massaging this is good for the lungs and heart. The zu lan li is on the channel related to the stomach. This is good to massage for the digestive system, and also for treating many other diseases. This is a longevity point.

A story said about 200 hundrend years ago, someone asked an old Japanese farmer the secret of his longevity family (three generations were all over one hundred years old and healthy): they did moxibustion on the Zu San Li points each month from the first to the eighth.

32. WEIGHT LOSS GONG

This is not for people who have kidney disease or severe stomach problems. Choose the type you prefer, but the results can't be seen until at least two weeks of constant exercise. Later, a person can continue according to their own needs. Only do this exercise when you are hungry! There is no time limit.

Step A: Assume the standing meditation posture.

Step B: Inhale and exhale in an exaggerated fashion; inhale and exhale as strongly as possible, until you stick out your chest and until you hold in your stomach as much as you can.

Step C: Inhale and exhale 40 times. Then you won't feel hungry.

Step D: When feeling hungry again, do this 20 to 60 times.

After you do this exercise for five or six days, you may not feel too well. Don't worry; this is normal. If you can get over this uncomfortable day, and continue doing it, to the seventh day, your hunger drive will disappear. Then you may stop doing this qigong, and start your regular three meals, but continue doing Steps B and C.

Another type of weight loss gong takes about 15 minutes. Do it before meals.

Step A. Begin with the sitting posture, knees straight

at 90 degrees or less.

Step B. Form your hand into a fist, male with the right, female with the left.

Step C. Place the elbow on the knee (same side) and head on the fist; your head, knee, and foot should be aligned in one vertical line.

Step D. "Sigh" to breath out the waste qi first.

Step E. For one or two minutes, relax, imagining all worries, pressure and depressed feelings gone: you are happy.

Step F. Inhale freely, as deeply as you can, until your lower stomach sticks out like a frog. Then breath out all the dirty qi from inside your body totally through your mouth, slowly and softly, until your lower stomach holds back as much as it can.

Step G. Do this for seven to eight minutes, stop for a few seconds, then continue doing it for another seven to eight minutes.

A third type of weight loss gong:

You may do this exercise after you have finished the first or the second type, or you can do it alone.

Step A. Use the sitting meditation posture (you may also sit on a chair) and lower your head a little and smile.

Step B. Place your hands together: male left hand

on the right, female contrary, fingers apart a little, with middle fingers stretching and thumbs touching.

Step C. Count your breaths, eyes closed slightly.

Step D. Breath in through the nose very slowly to the chest, then exhale slowly. Do this for five minutes.

Step E. For another five minutes, breath in the natural way, slowly, evenly, and softly.

Step F. For another five minutes, just breath in your normal way. When your mind focuses on breathing, you will feel half-asleep.

Ending form: after you finish each of the above three exercises, keep quiet for a while, then slowly put both your hands on the chest to massage in circles, 18 times until your palms feel hot. Then use your fingers to comb through your hair, from forehead to the back, 18 times. Then dry wash your face to massage from forehead to chin and inward out, 18 times. Then stretch your arms up and exhale to sigh loudly.

33. RELIEF FROM TIREDNESS

Sleep helps you recover from physical tiredness, but it can't always relieve tiredness of the mind. As days go on, the mental exhaustion may accumulate and lead to sickness. Massaging the ears is one of the ways to relieve mental tiredness. It can also stop unpleasant movements of the stomach and bowels. Use your thumb, index, and middle fingers to rub the bottom of the ears hard until hot. Then pull the ears downward 12 times, then pull the same spots up hard 12 times.

34. ANOTHER WEIGHT LOSS GONG
By Li Jian-zhuo (Qigong Magazine, 2/95)

This gong will help you lose weight without going on a diet, but it will take a couple of years. You may do it once a day, either before going to bed, or an hour after the lunch. Massaging these points has not just helped me lose weight, but has benefited my health.

Step A: Massage the guan yuan point (four inches down the navel). This point, also known as the lower dan tian, gathers the qi, and can also adjust qi and blood. It is in charge of birth, and builds up health. Massage and press it 1,000 times (this will take about 15 minutes.)

Step B: Press and massage the tian shu point (3 inches on the sides of the navel), then the di wuan (3 inches above the navel), and then the zhong wuan (5 inches above the navel), each point for three to five minutes.

Step C: Later I added two more points: the yin jiao (1.5 inches below the navel), and the wai ling (1.5 inches below the tian shu), each three minutes.

35. QIGONG TREATMENT FOR DIABETES

No matter which one of the following forms you do,

use the same method of breathing: breathe through the nose with the mouth naturally closed, your tongue touching the maxilla, sending the qi down to the lower dan tian and holding it as long as you can. When you breathe out, let down your tongue. Repeat breathing in this way. At the same time, imagine a good thought: "Saliva has filled my mouth and is going to nourish my lungs." When your mouth has produced a lot of saliva, rinse your mouth, using your tongue to massage your mouth in a circle repeatedly. Then divide the saliva, swallowing it three times down into the lower dan tian.

1. Yin Shi Zi Xian Form:

a.) Start in the sitting posture with legs folded, wearing a casual dress or loose clothing.

b.) Place the back of the right hand on the left palm, close to the lower stomach, gently on the legs.

c.) Shake the body from left to right, seven to eight times. Straighten the body, nose, navel on one line, chin a little lowered. Breath out thoroughly and slowly through the mouth, then the tip of tongue touches the upper maxilla, and inhale through the nose slowly, evenly, three to seven times.

d.) Close your eyes and sit as long as you wish.

e.) After sitting meditation, breath out through the mouth ten times, then shake the body, and shoulders, and head. Slowly loosen the body, rubbing the top of the thumbs until hot, using them to rub the eyelids, nose, and sides of nose; rubbing the palms until hot, then rubbing the ears, head, chest, stomach, back, arms, legs, and bottom of the feet. Wait until the sweat has dried.

f.) Do this three or four times a day, 30-40 minutes each time. Usually after a month, your diabetes will improve; three to four months later, you may be cured. But you'll still have to continue the exercise for 20-30 minutes each day.

2. Hao Ran Form:

a.) Lie on either the left or the right side; your head should be on a shoulder-level pillow, chin lowered a little, eyes half closed, as if looking at the top of the nose slightly. With your mouth closed naturally, inhale through the nose. Gently put the palm of your upper hand on your hip, the other palm on the pillow, facing up, about four inches away from your head. The waist should be bent a little, the upper leg forming a 120-degree angle on the other leg, which is slightly bent. Keep the mind on the dan tian point and breath naturally.

b.) Lie on your back, head on a pillow, relaxed, breathing naturally, legs straight with toes upward, hands at the sides, mind on the dan tian.

c.) From a sitting posture, your body and legs should form a 90-degree angle, and keep your chin lowered a little. Place the palms on the knees, and keep the shoulders and arms relaxed. The nose, eyes, and mouth are in the same form as the lying-on-side posture. The mind is on the dan tian. Breathe as long, evenly, and softly as you can.

3. Ke Shang Form:

a.) Stand with your feet as wide as your shoulders, toes inward a little, curled to hold the ground, knees and hips slightly bent, eyes half closed, tongue touching the maxilla, the mind on the lower dan tian.

b.) Lift both hands slowly from the sides, to shoulder level, then slowly bend the elbows, moving the hands to the chest.

c.) Move your two fists from the chest, changing into a posture as if the hands were holding a ball, with fingers angled down, two shao shang points slightly touched.

d.) Breathe naturally until calm, then begin breathing in through the nose, breathing out through the mouth. At first, both the nose and mouth breathe in turns one at a time. Then separately breathe in two times (pause after half a breath, then continue in), then breathe out, until your breathing becomes smooth. Then breathe in three times at a time (pause at each one-third of a breath), and out one time. When breathing in, imagine sending the qi all the way down to the bottom of the lungs, to fill them; when breathing out, imagine the qi moving from the chest to the armpits, along the inner side of the arms and into the wrists, to the palms and out the tips of the thumb and index finger.

e.) Repeat the exercise. When saliva fills your mouth,

imagine sending it down like water, to nourish your lungs when you swallow it.

f.) To end the form, the mind gathers qi in the dan tian, then both hands slowly move down to the lower dan tian, then massage the chest, the sides of the chest, and loosen the shoulders and forearms.

36. THE SECRETLY PASSED GONG

From the standing posture, relax the shoulders and elbows. Circle the arms slowly up from the sides and then to the front and hold the palms together in front of your chest. The fingertips should be angled up (like in Buddhist worship). Then point the fingertips forward, a little higher than the navel. Turn the left hand on the top, pull the left elbow backward, and with the two hands draw a parallel circle at the left side of the body, the right forearm against the left side body.

After drawing the circle, move both hands back to the front. Then turn the right hand on the left palm, pull the right elbow backward, and draw a circle, the left forearm against the right side of the body. Then both hands move back to the front. Repeat the left-right exercise 24 times.

To end the form, return to the beginning posture - two palms together holding in front of the chest for a while. Then spread apart the small fingers, the next fingers, then the middle, then the index fingers, and the thumbs. Press with the index finger (left for men, right for women) on the cheng jiang point below the lower lip.

37. KE XIA GONG

From a standing posture, feet parallel and as wide as the shoulders, toes holding the ground, knees and waist slightly bent, relax. Eyes should be half closed, the tongue up touching the maxilla. Move both hands slowly from the sides to the lower dan tian, left hand over the right. Breathe naturally at first, and keep the mind on the dan tian, until you feel your palms feeling warm. Then began to inhale deeply, down to the dan tian, letting the qi fill the lower stomach and stay there.

When inhaling, hold your bottom and lower stomach. Do this for 15-20 minutes.

To end the form, slowly open your eyes and bring both hands slowly back to the sides. Shake the four limbs and relax.

Do the exercises, and choose the proper diet to assist. After a certain time, depending on how you feel, you may reduce the pills you have been taking, or even stop taking them.

38. HERE ARE SIX SPECIFIC WAYS TO USE MEDITATION TO TREAT DISEASES:

a.) Focus the mind on the lower dan tian to treat upper chest pain (bloated feeling), pain on the sides of the chest, back pain, shoulder pain, heart pain, coughing, or when your upper body feels hot and your lower body feels cold. (dan tian shown on the chart)

b.) Focus the mind on the zu san li to treat pain. If this does not help, focus the mind on the bottom wrinkle of the toes. (zu san li point is on the chart)

c.) Focus the mind on the place between the feet to treat headache, red eyes, hot mouth, acute lower stomach pain, or stiff neck.

d.) For waist or foot pain, imagine a ten-foot hole in front of you and visualize the bottom of it.

e.) Focus your mind directly on the sick spot. It is best to have knowledge of the five elements in order to get the best results.

f.) Focus your mind on the top of the head if the body feels heavy and haggard or the skin itches.

39. THE SIX WAYS OF BREATHING OUT BENEFIT AND EXERCISE DIFFERENT ORGANS:

a.) "huh" is exercising the heart

b.) "shu" is for the liver

c.) "xi" is for the san jiao (a Chinese medicine term refers to the upper, middle and lower part of the body. You may see it on the chart.)

d.) "ss" is to exercise the lungs

e.) "hu" for exercising the spleen and stomach

f.) "chwee" is for the kidneys

For Qigong Teachers and Healers

CHAPTER 14

Qigong teachers must be loving and caring, and have the knowledge and ability to help students and solve problems.

Qi treats diseases, and if the psychological aspects and beliefs are taught, qi will work even better. So a teacher should always encourage and tell students positive messages and stories, like the many well-known masters do.

Here is a story about how a doctor cured his patient. The famous ancient Chinese doctor, Zhang Zhongjing, was also a qigong master. He had a hunch one of his patients was suffering from a psychosomatic illness. She believed that she had swallowed a fly; since then, she had suffered a sick stomach. So he secretly put a dead fly in the food that she had thrown out. Zhang showed her the fly and told her she had thrown the fly out. And the woman believed it and got well.

Pay attention to different individuals and their reactions: the way of understanding and the ability of each student to learn is different. So is their health. But to all, the general rule is the same: the mouth should be closed slightly, they should breathe through the nose, relax the shoulders, waist, and lower stomach, and think of (but not too focus too heavily on) qi gathering in the lower Dan Tian. All movements should be relaxed.

If a student has just finished a difficult exercise, tell the student to breathe out hard through nose a few times. Then there should be no problem continuing to do qigong.

A teacher should know that different people do

meditation differently – I don't mean the form, but the nature, the mind. Some students are active, sensitive, and some are quiet. Help them according to their nature.

The following are some methods:

1. When doing sitting meditation, you should do some exercise first to prepare the students. The steps:

a.) Place palms on knees and crouch down; turn clockwise and counter-clockwise, each 20 times.

b.) Stand up, then crouch down, repeating 20 times.

c.) Place the left foot somewhat in back, so the leg is stretched, then squat on the right heel like a lunge, three times. Change the legs and repeat three times. Change and repeat for 10 times total.

d.) Stand and lift heels off the ground, 20 times.

e.) Sit on the floor with the knees out, the bottoms of the feet touching at center. Hold the toes and use the elbows to press the knees, down and up 20 times.

f.) Sitting on the floor, bring the left foot to the right thigh (or close to the right leg). Hold the left foot with the right hand, and with the left hand press the left knee, 20 times. Then change to the other. Gradually make the knee touch the floor.

g.) Fold the right leg at 90 degrees, with the right side of the foot on the floor, on the middle line of the body or even further to the left. Then try to move the left foot onto the right thigh. Press the left knee down; the best is to touch the floor. Then change to the other leg and repeat. Practice for a long time, and your students will be prepared for the exact posture for sitting meditation.

Keep in mind that usually the students can't sit for a long time. They need to develop patience and persistence to practice.

After the training, you may guide the students to shake their ankles, massage the knees, turn their waists and shake their legs, then place the hands close to lower Dan Tian, and rest for a while.

2. To those who become anxious because the result has not been obvious, guide them to follow the rules; if a person works only on being nice first, then he can relax.

3. An important way to avoid problems is to teach the students the correct, fundamental concepts and ideas about qigong, and some knowledge of it. To those who have problems, judge what is the cause first, so as to suit the remedy to the case. First of all, tell the student to repeat in his mind, "Slow down." He may cough, press his Ren Zhong point for a few seconds, and beat his chest slightly, or someone else can help do these things.

4. There are ways to help schizophrenic and mentally ill patients, but they must learn a special type of qigong. That subject will not be included in this book. There are some qigong hospitals in China for such of patients, but not in the United States. So you may not want to accept students who have that history or genetic

heredity. The best way to find out is to ask the student directly. You can also check their eyes: the way they look at people is different.

Or check their hands, looking for some sign that can tell you about the mental well being. There will be another book in which a chapter will talk about it. Suffice to say that if you cannot help them, do not try, but help direct them to help elsewhere.

5. If a student is suddenly shocked by something while doing meditation, tell him to be calm, to slowly open his eyes, and to inhale deeply. Take a walk for a while, with the mind on the lower Dan Tian. When he is calm, continue.

6. Always give guidance gently. Speak softly near the meditating student.

7. When qi stuck somewhere, usually it is caused by the body not being relaxed, or the mind too nervous, or the breathing too uneven. Then the student may feel a stuffy stomach, a chest that is suffocating and hot, constipation, thirst, agitation, etc. The way to solve this is to tell him to massage his stomach, counterclockwise, circling from small gradually into bigger, at the same time pressing his chest lightly and mind picturing that the stuffy qi goes down along the legs and into the Yong Quan points (bottom of feet).

8. If the problem is caused by qi going the wrong way, it is because the student did not guide it properly, or had his mind on a certain point in the wrong way. Either he was thinking too hard and too focused on a point, or

108

he was shocked by something. The student may feel the chest tightening, the stomach sick, the heart beating faster, etc. The way to solve this is to tell him to place both palms facing each other in front of his chest, and push and pull but not touch each other, breathing naturally, with the mind picturing that the stuffy qi is led out when the hands are pulling. Then bring both hands to the sides, slowly lift to the armpits, and inhale, with no mind work. Slowly the hands should move down along the sides of the legs, the mind imagining the shocked qi goes down to the bottom of the feet and down into the earth, three feet deep.

9. The teacher can also use acupoints to treat problems. If the student's head feels heavy, numb, swollen, and painful, usually it is caused by mind focusing too hard. The way to treat this is to fold four fingers lightly into a half fist. Point the thumb at the Bai Hui point, and use qi to push and at the same time twist a half circle. This method can be used on some other points, too.

10. If the student loses control of his spontaneous movement, for example the head turning (he can't stop it by himself), the teacher may put both middle fingers lightly into his ear holes (listening acupoints), circling around gently and making a vibration. Then suddenly pull out the fingers; his ears will hear a thunder-like sound. The problem usually will be solved.

11. If the student feels his qi running up and down on sinister errands, the teacher may use a qi "sword" - index and middle fingers pointing at the Que Pen acupoint (the concave part of the scapula). Vibrate the "sword"

for a while, then suddenly turn over the wrist as if the fingers are turning the big tendons on the scapula's concave face. Then the problem can be solved.

12. If the student feels his back and chest are extremely hot, or frozen cold, use the thumb and the index finger to point at the Xin Yu point (one inch away from the fifth vertebra) and the Ge Yu point (one inch from the seventh joint of the spine). Pull and shoot back, repeating three or four times. His problem should be solved.

13. If the student feels lower stomach swelling with qi and feels uncomfortable, use thumbs and index fingers to hold the muscles on both sides four to five inches from the navel. Pull them, at the same time turning the fingers. When you hear the sound from the stomach, the problem is solved.

14. To correct the student from falling asleep when meditating, use middle fingers in the ear holes until he wakes up and makes some sound. Another way is to use the middle fingers to point at both Ja Che points, first vibrating the fingers with palms facing downward, then suddenly turning the palms up, then down again, up and down several times within a minute, until the student makes a sound. Then point at his Er Ya point (1.5 inches from the corner of the mouth), using the finger to point and "knock" (without touching) for a few times. The student will wake up.

15. If a student feels the whole body is so hot he can't take it anymore, the teacher may use the qi sword fingers to point at his Da Zhui point, to guide and push

the hot qi down the spine, 10-20 times.

16. If someone is bent over or down too much and can't control himself, use the thumbs and four fingers to hold the big tendons of the shoulders, twisting at the same time. The tendon will make a sound. The problem should be solved.

17. If the student keeps shaking his shoulders and has lost control of his movements, use your thumbs and four fingers hold the big tendons of the shoulders. Lift first, then twist three to five times, then with the thumbs massage the Da Zhui, then push at the same time massaging the muscles on the sides of the spine. Also knock as if playing a piano. After three to five times the problem will be solved.

18. If someone's hands are waving and he has lost control, wait until his arms come down. Use the thumb and index finger hold the muscle on the Qu Chi point; lift up, and right away hold the He Gu point's fine tendon, pulling and twisting. You must start with the right hand first, then the left, because the lung qi is related to the right hand. If you calm it first, it will be easier to calm the left.

19. Someone may lose control of the movement of his waist. Use both thumbs and index fingers hold the Tian Cheng points (at inside tops of the ears). Lift first, then loosen, repeating three to five times. Then use the thumbs, vibrating on the Lu Lu Guan point (the fourteenth joint of the spine) lightly. Soon the problem will be solved.

111

20. Some male students may have a problem holding the qi. He will feel the qi drain from the Hui Yin point (directly underneath the bottom), and someone may have a little emission. Ask him to lie down, and use sword fingers to give qi treatment to the Qi Zhong and Guan Yuan points, until he feels his stomach slightly warm. He will needs some treatments, but his problem can be solved.

21. Some male student may have another problem; his penis is hard all the time, even when he sleeps. The teacher may use thumb and middle finger to hold both the Lao Gong and He Gu points to give qi treatment. After some treatments, the problem will be solved.

Drawings of Some Channels and Acupoints

CHAPTER 15

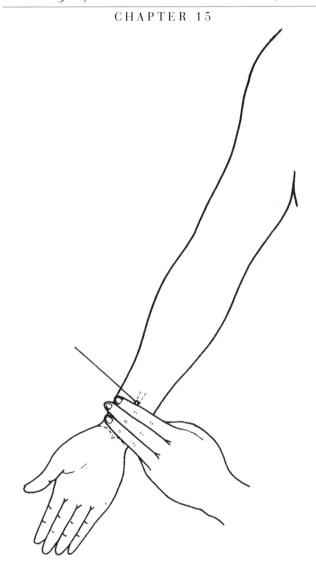

HOW TO FIND NEI GUAN

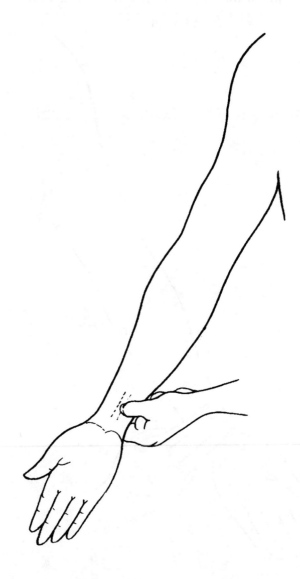

MASSAGE NEI GUAN

By Yanling L. Johnson

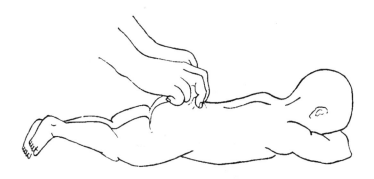

THE WAY TO MASSAGE A BABY

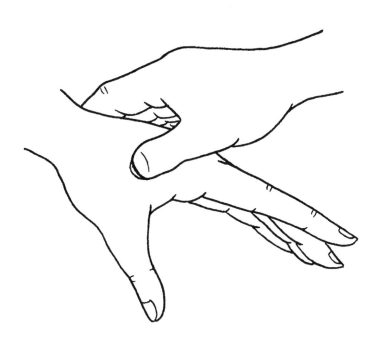

MASSAGE HE GU

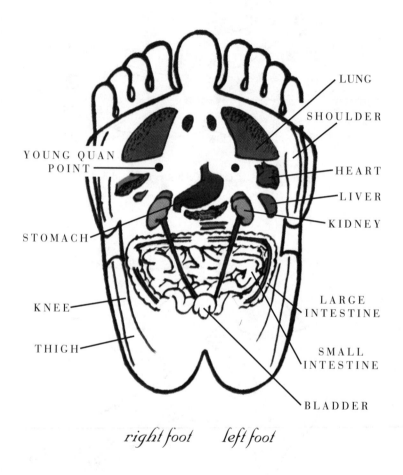

right foot   *left foot*

MASSAGE POINTS IN THE FEET

116

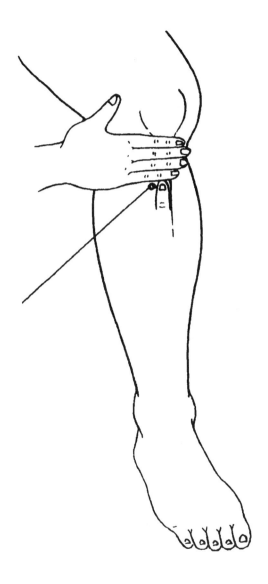

ZU SAN LI

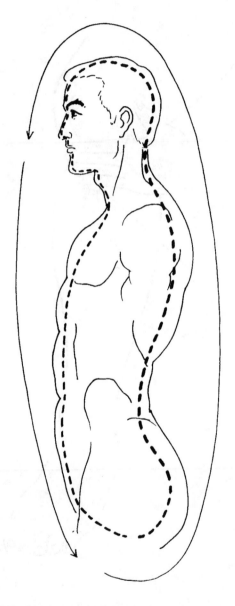

THE SMALL CIRCULATION OF QI

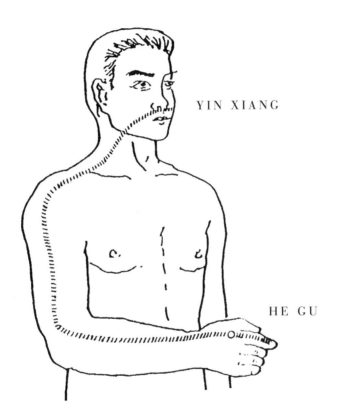

YIN XIANG

HE GU

WHEN MASSAGE HE GU

Herbal Cooking Tips

CHAPTER 16

By the time a doctor can diagnose a disease, the disease has already made its move. The doctor is only treating something that has already happened – and he can't always stop further progression of the disease. When the symptom shows, the disease has started and has been growing inside the body for a long time – one year, ten years, many years. It takes more than one day for water to form a block of ice.

This is why it always takes time, maybe a long time, to treat disease and recover – and mainly it is the body which must heal itself. If the doctor uses a certain chemical to "cure" the disease, the side effects of the chemical will at the same time harm some of the patient's organs. One time we went to visit a friend and saw him take over ten different drugs given by his doctor, to "treat" his lung problem. Later appeared kidney problems. I felt sorry for him, but could not say much. I told my husband, "The doctor will kill my friend soon, believe me." A half year later, my friend left the world – he had become in my eyes another victim of too many drugs. For some acute diseases, drugs may be necessary as an immediate measure, but not for the long-term treatment.

In our lives there are too many chemicals already: so many chemicals in drinking water that you can smell it. There are chemicals in our drinks, in our food, in our grains, in our clothing, in our medicine cabinets, under our sinks, in our houses...in the air. It is scary to think of how a baby grows up among chemicals, taking them in and silently being affected by them.

We spring forth from the natural world. The less chemicals that we use and take, the better for us. We can make our own decisions about how we wish to live, and make the best out of our food.

Nowadays people have become more aware of the side effects of drugs. They have developed a concern about what they eat and want to take their health in to their own hands. Organic food has become more popular.

Eating the right food, and using organic food, can prevent future diseases, help to treat diseases, and help you maintain your health.

As your body changes, and as the seasons change, to eat meals and use herbs in an adaptable way is the art and wisdom of Chinese medicine. I will have another book solely on this subject.

Now let us talk about herbs. Both food and herbs can perform functions that the Western laboratory has not yet proven. For example, from the dry plant of coptis chinensis, the Western lab extracts chemicals that kill germs. In Chinese culture ("unscientific", according to Western medicine) this plant has been used for treating three parts of the body by processing it in three different ways: steamed, cooked in honey, and raw.

Herbal cooking has started gaining attention. Yet one herb does not suit all. A person should not drink the herbal tea or herbal wine or take the herb only because of an advertisement, or because other people say it is good. Each person's body has its own needs. For example, ginseng is good, but not good for all people; garlic is good, but not suitable to some patients who have certain disease. Don't drink just any herbal tea; it must be the right kind for you.

The Chinese tea is all right. The Chinese, all Chinese, have been drinking tea for some five thousand years. If it were bad, it would not have lasted.

However, herbs work slowly and gradually, but gently working on the "root". It takes time and patience to see the results. If someone excepts a sudden change, then forget my book and maybe go get some chemicals.

The following tips may help you in some way make the right decision. Use the proper herbs in cooking, so as to benefit your health.

Let food be our health-care taker. Here are some tips:

1. TEA

I am not talking about the herbal tea here, but the common teas. Herbal tea may be good for some people, but bad to others, depending on their needs. Generally there are three types of tea: green tea, which contains the most Vitamin C after being dry roasted, jasmine tea, and woolong (or spelt as OOlong, a dark tea).

Common tea can be the daily drink for almost everyone: old and young, even little children, who can rinse their mouths after eating. This will help prevent tooth decay. Use the soaked tea leaves to wipe the baby's mouth to treat ulcers. Don't worry about the tea stain, it is easy to brush off.

Tea is good for treating diarrhea; it can neutralize and release some poisons. It helps to relieve drunkenness because it can neutralize some of the alcohol.

A patient who has uremia has to be careful about tea. Don't drink tea before going to bed – especially if you have some sleep disorder. It is better not to drink tea with an empty stomach. All the teas aid in digestion, especially after eating meat or a greasy meal.

You just have to learn how to make tea in the proper way, and learn how to drink it.

Don't leave the tea leaves in the hot water for over six minutes. The best time is about three minutes. The water should be boiling. Then wait for a minute, then pour it into the tea pot. If it is a tea bag, a minute should be long enough.

If you are making green tea, note that the color, when finished, will be quite light. If you try to make it as dark as the other teas, it will be too strong. Green tea's taste is delicate.

All the teas will refresh your mind, and, although they contains some tea tannins and caffeine, (much less than coffee), they contain nutrients like Vitamin C, amino acids, and others good things.

2. GINGER

Fresh ginger, green onion, garlic, wine, and vinegar are all good herbs as well as important spices in Chinese cooking. If we know how to use them in the right way, it will not only bring out the best flavor (and get rid of the smell of fish and mutton) but benefit health.

Ginger - also named Jiang in Chinese - has been both an herb and a spice since ancient time in Chinese culture. As an herb, the hidden meaning of "Jiang" is "the battlefield", because it is against "a hundred heresies". As an herb, it's good to eat often, but not too much at a time; it won't be good to your eyes, nor to the patient who has piles. It is good when someone is catching cold suddenly, for it will bring the cold out of the pores. It is good for treating a sick stomach, dizziness, and rapid heart-beat. Like garlic and green onion, ginger also kills germs.

As a spice, it can make meat tender and prevent the oil or fat from smelling putrid. When cooking meat or seafood, putting some fresh ginger in can make them more tasty and benefit your health. To cook crab with some sliced ginger can balance the yin and yang between the two foods.

It is good to eat ginger more often in summer, but not in autumn.

Recipes:

a.) Put sliced fresh ginger in boiling or hot water with brown sugar, Chinese dates (each 30 gm). Drink as tea. The drink treats PMS caused by lack of blood and chi.

b.) Sliced ginger boiled with just brown sugar can be drunk when hot or warm (when it is cool, it is okay, too, but the warmer kind results better and faster). It will warm you, warding off colds and headaches caused by dampness.

c.) For body odor under the armpits, use fresh ginger to rub that place often and it will be cured.

d.) When cooking chicken or other meat, or fish, crab, or shrimp, put sliced fresh ginger (or together with green onion) with them. It can bring out the flavor of the food and make it more tasty. The amount is flexible, depending on the taste you like.

3. GREEN ONION

It benefits the lungs, smooths the yang, releases poisons, helps swelling. It is good to treat a cold, too. When stir fried, cook it in the oil first, then put the other ingredients in. The stock is the good part, the longer and bigger the better.

It is not good to eat with honey or dates.

4. GARLIC

Everyone knows it kills germs. It also strengthens the stomach, unblocks stagnancy, releases the poison caused by eating bad crab or being bit by bugs. It prevents flu. It prevents cancer. It prevents heart disease. We are talking about fresh garlic, not those powdered and dry garlic products. They are far from good.

It is not good to eat too much a time, neither is it good to eat too much of it in March. It is not good to eat it in conjunction with raw fish. It is not good for people who have athlete's feet or seasonal diseases.

As a spice, it is good for cooking with vegetables and fish.

Recipes:

a.) Salad dressing: Put the dark kind of vinegar, some soy sauce, a little sesame oil, and mashed garlic together. Flavor to your own taste. Poue over the salad. The dressing makes sliced cucumber very tasty, too.

b.) For fried dishes: Just fry in the oil first. When the garlic flavor comes out, put in the vegetables or fish.

c.) Put pealed garlic in the water together with some other spices and with the fish.

5. LING ZHI

This mushroom has been considered a longevity herb for thousands of years in China. It can be soaked in wine for two weeks, to drink a little daily.

Here is one recipe:

Ling Zhi and Sweet Rice Soup

It is helpful for menopause. Use ling zhi, sweet rice (each 50 gm), and some sugar. Wash the ingredients; cut the ling zhi into small pieces and put them in a cotton fabric bag. (They may be cooked whole too.) Cook the two ingredients in a clay or glass pot with 2.5 cups of water at a low temperature. Simmer until the rice is done. Add sugar to taste. Once a day, after seven days, you'll see the result.

It can be a long term diet, and benefit health.

Sweet rice strengthens the spleen. The soup nourishes the heart, benefits the kidneys, builds against weakness. It also treats the distracted mind.

6. PONG DA HAI

Use for sore throat. To make tea: use four pong da hai in a cup and pour in boiling water. Wait until the seeds open. Drink daily. This will soothe throat pain, and benefit lung qi.

However, there are different causes of sore throat. This recipe is for coughing caused by burning sensations in the lungs. Pang da hai also helps smooth liver qi.

7. LYCIUM (GOU JI ZI)

In I Ching, there is an ancient poem that says, "Travel a thousand miles, take lycium everyday." It builds up the liver and kidneys and benefits the eyes. You may put it in soup or dishes. It can be used to make tea, or be made into herbal wine. To make the herbal wine, take 30 gm or more and soak it in wine for a week or two. Drink a little (about three teaspoons) each day.

8. YI REN RICE

Yi ren rice is my favorite grain and herb. It helps lose weight in a nice way - by getting rid of body waste and extra water. It makes the skin younger and smoother. It stops the cancer cells from growing. It strengthens the spleen, nourishes the lungs. And it is easy to cook. You may cook it in soup or in rice. Or make the rice dish every day. Each time use 30 gm or more.

9. SHAN YAO

Shan yao is favorite food for many Chinese. It nourishes the spleen, lungs, and kidneys. There are fresh kinds (which are so expensive here), but you can get the dry kind in the herbal store, too. The dry shan yao is much cheaper. Soak the dry herb in water until it becomes soft, then cook into soup. Use 30 gm or more. You may cook it with other food, too. You can eat it daily.

10. LONG GAN
(THE CHINESE WORD ARE: THE DRAGON'S EYES)

Fresh long gan is a wonderful fruit. The dry kind can be found both in the herbal store or in the Chinese grocery store. It nourishes the heart and spleen, and helps with sleeplessness, forgetfulness. It benefits qi.

11. BLACK SESAME SEEDS

They benefit the eyes and blood, and build up energy. They are good to the liver and kidneys. Roasted them and eat whatever way you like. Use 30 gm or more.

12. MONG BEAN

Its soup clears summer heat and poison.

13. SALT

It clears heat, cools blood, releases poison and helps with vomit.

14. VINEGAR

Vinegar kills germs. It helps get rid of coagulated blood after a woman gives birth. It helps digest. As a spice, it kills germs in fish, meat, and vegetables, and brings out flavor. But don't eat it with other herbs or drugs. It is better for a woman to have more than for a man. It is not good to eat too much at a time because it will harm the stomach.

15. BEI MU RICE SOUP

For treating bronchus and lungs. Ten gm bei mu (powder is better), 50 gm brown rice, plus some rock sugar (optional). Put bei mu powder into boiling, cooked rice soup. Then turn it all down to a low temperature let it boils for two or three minutes until the soup is done. Eat both in the morning and evening.

16. PEANUT RICE SOUP

Use 30 gm raw peanuts plus 100 gm rice. Cook together, and eat both in the morning and in the evening on an empty stomach. It nourishes yang energy, especially good for male.

17. RAW PEANUT SOUP

This benefits the lungs. Use 150 raw peanuts, and cook with some rock sugar until soft. Drink and eat daily.

It nourishes qi and the yin energy of the lungs, and helps with coughing and shortness of breath.

18. FRUIT

Go with the season and eat more fruit from the farm.

In summer eat more watermelon (but quit when autumn starts); it helps clear heat and poisons from your body.

a.) Pear: It is good to clear the heat and phlegm.

b.) Apricots: It is not good to eat too many apricots at a time. They may cause nose bleeds. Nor should you eat too many plums at a time.

c.) Oranges: Oranges and tangerines are good. Tangerines' white pitch cooked with rock sugar helps clean phlegm. Use the skin of the tangerine and its pitch to make tea; it helps reduce gas in the stomach.

d.) Apple: The apple is good to the spleen and stomach.

e.) Banana: It is good for clearing heat (making your body feel cool) and moist bowels. They will unblock the blood qi channel.

f.) Lemon: Lemon buts thirst and summer heat. It calms during pregnancy.

g.) Grapes: They benefits blood qi, strengthen the tendons and bones, help urination.

h.) Pomegranates : They produce saliva, kill worms, and help cure dysentery.

i.) Luo han guo: It helps to clear the lungs and moist bowels, and clears phlegm and sore throat caused by summer heat.

j.) Pineapple: It helps clear heat and solve thirst. It aids in digestion and stops loose bowels.

k.) Peach: It nourishes qi and produce saliva, moving blood.

l.) Water chestnuts (the fresh kind is better): They help produce saliva, clear phlegm, and clear the eyes.

m.) Coconut meat: It builds up consumptive weakness and kills worms.

n.) Chinese dates: They nourish the Zhong-benefit qi, build up the blood, and calm the mind.

19. NUTS AND SOME GRAINS

a.) Chestnuts: They benefit the spleen, stomach and kidneys, stimulate blood circulation and also help stop bleeding.

b.) Sweet apricot seeds: They moistens the lungs and calms asthma. You may cook it in water or rice soup, or eat it roasted. Its bitter kind has other herbal functions.

c.) Roasted sesame seeds (the black kind is better): They help get rid of stomach gas. For patients who have had an operation on the breathing organs, white seeds are better. For those who are weak or suffer from lack of nutrition, black seeds are good. Chew and eat them three times a day before meals.

d.) Lotus seeds: They nourish the body and benefit qi; they are good to treat many diseases. You may use them to cook with rice, with chicken, and together with dates, walnuts, long gan, etc.

e.) Walnut: It builds up the kidneys and strengthens the waist. It helps with seminal emission, asthma, and moist bowels.

20. BANYAN TREE FLOWER

Use the red/light brown kind and cook it in two big bowls of water with a little rock sugar. Cook it down until just one bowl is left. Get rid of the solids and drink the liquid. It treats cold, diarrhea, and mild poisons.

21. VEGETABLES

a.) The xianggu mushroom: It helps build up qi and benefit the stomach; it also releases the poison caused by smallpox. It is good for diabetes and cancer patients.

Other mushrooms benefit the intestines and stomach, encourage regular qi, and clear phlegm.

b.) Spinach: It is good to eat cooked -- cook it in soup, or stir fry it for a very short time. It is good to cook with tofu and both will benefit health even better.

c.) Radish: It is good for the lungs. If you are coughing a lot and have phlegm, put some tea leaves and white radish with some ginger, and cook in water until the radish is mushy. You may also put a little salt in the tea. Drink twice a day.

d.) Seaweed: All seaweed help clear the heat, release extra fluid from the body, and soften scrofula.

22. MEAT

a.) Lamb: It is good to eat more in the winter but not in summer, because it builds up yang.

b.) Chicken: It is good because it warms the zhong, benefits qi, and builds up energy. It fortifies a mother's milk when she is breast feeding.

c.) Pheasant meat: It builds up the zhong and liver, benefits qi, is good for the eyes, and is good for people having a weak spleen and stomach. But it is not good to eat together with chicken.

d.) Bone: Its soup has always been important in Chinese cooking. Use any beef, pork, or other meat bones. Cook them in water until it becomes milky, and save it in a big glass jar and use it to cook noodles, to make vegetable soup, or even to make rice. It is much better than taking calcium pills. You can always get rid of the fat when you use it (leave the jar in the refrigerator and the fat will be hardened). By the way, a little fat from the marrow is good for you.

e.) Meat skins: In American culture, people throw all skin away when eating. Fish skin, which is so tasty, contains much nutrition. A certain kind of donkey skin in Chinese medicine is a special, nutritious herb. Even eat some pork skin once in a while to benefit your health. I remember my mother told me when I was little, "Eat some, it helps you grow shiny hair!" To cook it and make it tasty, you just put ginger, green onion, soy sauce, and a little cooking wine with water. You can also put in some other spices, such as a little "five spice".

f.) Kidney: Many people worry only about choles-terol, in a negative way - avoid it. But there is much to be pursued in the foods we eat. Animal organs can provide important parts of a diet. They all are like good herbs. Kidney will build up your kidneys, stop you from sweat-ing at night, prevent seminal emission, and provide re-lief from a certain type of lower back pain.

g.) Pork lung: Cook it with fresh lemon juice. It helps with constant coughing, when the phlegm is white and thin, and the chest feels stuffy. Use 15 gm lemon juice with 200 gm pork lung, and add a little salt. Cook it in water with salt and ginger and green onion. Eat the lung and drink the soup.

23. TOFU

Tofu is easy to digest and nutritious, and has been an important food for over two thousand years. In China there are tens of kinds of tofu products. Yet if someone eats it daily without other food containing calcium, the person's bones will become weak. Tofu lacks calcium.

Tofu is plain, so it is good to go with many flavors – you may cook it with meat, fish, or vegetables; or you may eat it "raw". Simply put some spices, or simply chopped green onion in it with a little salt and sesame oil.

24. FERMENTED SOYBEANS (BLACK COLOR)

Fermented soybean is a spice in Chinese cooking, yet a good herb, too. For a stomach that feels clogged up, and very uncomfortable (so as leading to get sick), cook the fermented soybeans with fresh ginger. Drink the soup.

For Mothers and Babies

CHAPTER 17

I began to be concerned about this subject after I saw some young mothers walking around in the cold grocery store just days after they gave birth. They had their delicate, newborn babies with them – to a place full of many people, and even more germs. Then I saw a TV show meant to teach young mothers how to take care of their newborns. I thought, "I must write what I know about what I learned from Chinese mothers - there are many good tips."

1. FOR MOTHERS

Mothers who have just given birth need to take good care of themselves in order to avoid future illness. When you are young, it seems something does not bother you and your body can recover quickly from problems. But it does not mean the problem has been caused – it may hide and grow quietly and wait until the right time, or when you become weak, or when you are aged. Then it comes out happily, one by one with others, to show you its power! That is why you should learn to take care of your health when you are young. Someone who wears shorts in cold weather to show how sexy her or his legs are will have knee problems in later years.

In Chinese culture, the time of child-bearing is a very important period in a mother's life. During the month after giving birth, she might contract a life-long disease, which can only be cured during another child's birth period. It may be very hard to cure.

Her nutrition is extremely important. Even a poor Chinese family would do their best to feed the mother best. The mother should stay in bed more, and avoid heavy labor, because "when a woman gives birth, all the joints of her body are opened", according to an old Chinese mothers' saying. It is true that it is easy to get arthritis if the mother catches cold during that month, which may show right away or later, in back pain, shoulder pain, etc.

And the mother does need rest; even the Chinese government gives its female employees fifty-six days' leave after the woman gives birth. It will take at least a month for the mother to recover. (According to another old Chinese mothers' saying, it will take a hundred days for the mother's bones to totally return to the original position.) Lying in bed will help the uterus recover sooner. The mother should always keep her body dry and warm, especially the joints. Even in hot weather, at night, she should keep a shirt on.

During that first month after giving birth, the mother's food should be more nutritious, so the mother will regain the blood that she lost giving birth. Also consider the needs of the baby if the mother is breast feeding.

First of all, during the month, never drink cold drinks; drink no carbonated pop or soda at all. The drink and food should not be too hot, either; just warm. Food should be cooked and easy to digest. Chicken and its soup and eggs are always important. Liver helps build up the blood. It can be delicious if you cook it with a little cooking wine (or any wine), soy sauce, ginger, and green onion. Sometimes if you like more flavor, put in a little five spice, or Chinese ba jiao (also called da liao).

Eat some variety of food, like fish and red meat. Ribs must cooked soft.

Bone soup is good for both the mother and baby.

Pork feet soup, cooked with only ginger, and green onion, and no salt, will make the mother's milk plentiful and of good quality.

Each day take a sip (two teaspoons) of herbal wine (the huang jiu wine is especially good for getting rid of a cold from the joints for a mother giving birth; it is gentle, too). You may drink it with a little honey, since honey helps release poison. But don't feed your newborn baby too much honey; it may cause the baby to have loose bowels, because honey belongs to the cool kinds of herbs. So a breast feeding mother should not eat too much honey, either. The saying is, "whatever the mother eats, the baby eats too."

The mother can also consult an acupuncturist to get to know her body better, and to get certain herbs cooking with the food for her needs, because each individual may need something more than just nutrition.

2. FOR BABIES

Never dress the baby in clothing that is too warm. If the baby's forehead is sweating, reduce the baby's clothes until you feel baby's palms are just lightly warm.

Baby's palms can always tell the mother if she or he is doing fine. Feel the baby's palm often to test the temperature. If the baby's hands are cold, the baby may need a little more clothing, or may have some stomach problem caused by cold. If the baby's hands are hot, the baby may need a little less clothing, or the mother may have fed the baby too much and the baby is having a digestion problem.

Take the baby out in the fresh air often. Choose a sunny, warm, no wind area after the baby is one month old. Begin with five or ten minutes, and gradually build to a longer time – no longer than 20 minutes. Be careful to never sunburn your baby.

Don't use synthetic diapers – many of them contain chemicals and they harm the baby's health, especially a female baby. Use only diapers that are pure cotton, with no other chemicals of any kind. If you can not find them, you will have to work more for the sake of your child: Worn out, soft pure cotton tee-shirts can make substitute "diapers" that you can use. The older and softer the better, you do not want to damage the baby's tender, delicate skin. Always keep the baby's bottom dry.

Massage your baby's feet – it helps the baby's digestion. They baby's digestive system is weak. Not feeding well, or in the wrong way, or with the wrong food will cause the baby problems.

Some babies may keep crying, day and night, some may have a facial color that does not look healthy, some throw up a lot or have diarrhea, or sweat a lot, or lose hair, etc. When such problems happen, they are usually caused by bad digestion, and the baby's spleen and stomach are in trouble.

In such cases, feed the baby less food but a little warm plain water, keep the baby's stomach warm. There are herbal formula only for babies in the herb store, or you may consult an experienced acupuncturist to get some herbs. You may also treat your baby to gentle massage.

Treatment steps:

a.) You may massage gently the baby's lower stomach around the navel with four fingers, clockwise for three to five minutes, until the skin is a little red. Massage lightly at first, gradually adding a little strength.

b.) This step can also be used on a healthy baby once in a while, to prevent problems. Lay the baby on his or her stomach; use your index and middle finger from the top of the spine, on both sides of the spine, to go slowly down to the tail bone. Do this three to five times.

c.) Use the thumbs and index and middle fingers to knead and massage the skin along the sides of the spine, three to five times. This can also use on a healthy baby.

Do the treatment twice a day. Each treatment takes about ten minutes. Do it in a flexible way; judge the baby's case. Don't injure your baby's skin. Usually in less than a week your baby will get well.

There are three important points along the spine and if you are willing try this method, add this step:

Check the chart and find the points first. They are da chang (large intestine), wei yu (stomach), and pi yu (spleen) points. When your fingers move down and reach each point, you lift up the skin and pull; you may hear some sounds - then you are doing it right. It will not make your baby feel pain. Try it on yourself.

Now let's talk about how you feed your baby. I went to buy some baby food in jars, just to try them. I felt sorry for the babies, who are not able to tell their parents how bad the food tastes. Maybe there are some good kinds that I don't know. But there are so many ways your baby can eat better, more tasty, more nutritious food. Wouldn't you be glad is you could simply share your own food with your baby? Some real, good food? Of course you can't put food directly into your baby's mouth, but...

My experience is from observing my mother, an ordinary Chinese woman who raised her own children, her grandchildren, and a great granddaughter! She gained a reputation. When people around her found she was available, they often tried to get her to look after their babies.

When my daughter was two months old, my mother used a teaspoon to mix a little egg yolk with water (very thin). Then she fed my daughter, little by little. She would use a chopstick, dip it into vegetable soup, then put it into my daughter's mouth and say, "Let her prepare for the real food."

When my daughter was three months old, my mother mashed a quarter egg yolk into a little fried vegetable soup (no grease at all) and fed her. Two weeks later, she added the a third of the egg yolk, then half. When the baby five months old, my mother started to feed my baby one complete egg yolk in the soup. My mother told me, "The various kinds of the vegetable soup contain different nutrition. The baby's brains are growing, so feeding her a little egg yolk helps her grow brains better. But in the beginning you must be very careful, do not choke the baby." When my daughter was six months old, my mother always cooked rice (soft enough for a baby) with a little self-cooked (including liver, kidneys) broth, and easily-digested, cooked, mushy, vegetable leaves in a soup.

The following are some tips:

a.) Feed your baby some rice soup without rice in it as a drink. When your baby is four months old, feed him a little cooked, very mushy rice soup. Feed a little at first, then add a little more and observe. If the baby digests well, then add a little more. Half a baby food jar will be enough.

b.) The baby's diaper can always tell the parent if the child digests well, or has problems. When the baby's stool is mixed with some bits of milk and looks watery, the baby is having digestion problems. The mother should reduce the amount of food (not mother's milk) and feed the baby warm water until the stool becomes normal - a light brown, nicely thin or soft. If it looks green, the baby is catching cold. Keep the baby's stomach warm. (Even when your baby is healthy, and even in the hot weather when your baby is sleeping, you should always cover your baby's tummy with a piece of cotton material.) Feeding less baby food, but not your breast milk. Give more warm water only, and wait until the stools return to a normal color.

c.) Never feed the baby pop or soda – only water, with a little bit of sugar to bring to taste. Never feed your baby too much sugar.

All the cookies and cakes and drinks here contain too much sugar. If you go to China Town, you may find some cookies and cakes that do not contain as much sugar as you get from grocery stories.

d.) The baby who is not breast fed always needs

142

By Yanling L. Johnson

more water. Sometimes the baby may suffer from constipation; then feed the baby some water with a little honey
in it. Honey has some function to release the bowels, and
it works gently.

e.) A little fresh juice from fruit or vegetables will
be good to the baby. In spring, feeding your baby a little
fresh water chestnut juice helps your baby avoid disease.

f.) Always feed the baby at a regular hour, and in a
flexible way, and observe the baby's diaper – each baby
is different and has different needs.

My mother taught me all this knowledge, and I share
with you what I remember. Hopefully it will help some
young mothers to learn to take care of their babies.

The Natural Way for Remaining Beautiful

CHAPTER 18

You can take care of your own skin without chemicals. You can make it look younger and smoother, with fewer wrinkles, without using making up or having an operation. There are many methods of self-massage, and there are herbs you can use that will take care of your skin. You can make herbal tea, make herbal wine, or cook these herbs with your meals. Or you can make your own herbal lotion, etc. Acupuncture and qigong can also help.

Emotion and the health of your organs will affect your skin. All the options in this chapter will help you by helping with your organs. This will in turn improve your skin and help it look younger and more healthy.

A calm and peaceful mind, a relaxed and carefree mind is another a recipe for staying young.

1. SELF TREATMENT METHODS.

Self massage and exercise are safe and reliable. They all help with the blood qi circulation. You may choose one or two, or even all of them and do them daily.

a.) For wrinkles around the eyes

There are three acupoints around the eyes that can help you if you do the massage persistently. The two jing ming points are in the inside corners above your eyes at the deep area. The cheng qi points are down below the pupils and above the bone under your eyes. And the tong zi miu points are half an inch from the outside corners of your eyes, at the deep area on the temples. Press the jing ming with a little strength at first, five times, each time for one second. Then press the chen qi the same way, then the tong miu. The best time to do this is before you get up and before you go to bed.

b.) For staying healthy

Cut a large piece of fresh ginger, about 0.2 to 0.4 cm thick; use a needle to make some holes in it. Put it on your shen que point (navel) and light a moxa corn to heat the ginger. Every other day, heat the ginger on your navel until your skin feels hot and becomes lightly red. Usually you'll need three to five moxa for each treatment. (Pregnant woman are forbidden to use this method! Also patients who have had a fever during the night.)

You may buy mocssa from a Chinese herb store or in an acupuncture clinic.

c.) Face massage

Rub the hands together until hot, then massage your face like you are washing it. You may do this as many times, and for as long a time as you wish; the more the better. When massaging, your mouth should be closed, and you should breathe naturally and relax your body and mind.

d.) For staying healthy

Before getting up in the morning, gather your saliva and rinse inside your mouth until it is full in your mouth. Then swallow it all way down to lower dan tian. Then knock your teeth together 27 times.

e.) For the hair

Sit on the floor, legs straight and together, hands holding the lower legs and bend down your body until the top of your head touches your legs. Do this 12 times. Then move your feet apart, about fifteen inches from each other, and repeat, with the top of your head reaching down to touch the floor, another 12 times.

2. HERBAL RECIPES FOR FACIAL TREATMENT

You may go to a Chinese herbal store, or an acupuncture clinic to order these herbs, to ask them to make the recipe ingredients, or even make the formula.

a.) Ingredients:

Bai Zhi	250gm
Chuan Hong	250gm
Gua Lou Ren	250gm
Ji Gu Xian	150gm
Zao Jia	500gm
Da Dou	600gm
Chinese Red Beans	600gm.

Make the above into a powder, then mix with soya beans and Red Beans, and use it to wash the face everyday. The formula can last for a few months.

(Zao Jia has skin and threads, so dry it, get rid of them, and then you can make it into powder.)

b.) Ingredients:
   Dong Sang leaves.

Collect on a winter morning, the amount as you wish, and cook in water until thickened. When washing your face in the morning, put three tablespoons in the water and wash your face. It is very good to use in winter.

c.) Ingredients:

Tao Ren (rid of skin)	1 liter
Man Qing Zi	1 liter
Bai Shu	30gm
Tu Gua Gen	35gm
Wan Dou	2 liters.

Make the above into a powder and mix well, then use vinegar to make into a thick fluid. Keep it in a cool, dry place. Before using it to massage your face and hands, wash your face first. After washing, rinse it off with water. A hundred days later, your face will be smooth and shiny.

d.) Ingredients:

Lotus flower	35gm
lotus root	40gm
lotus seeds	45gm.

Dry all in shadow, then steam in a clay pot. Make into a powder and mix with light-colored honey. Divide it into balls (about as big as half of the soya bean). Take 15 gm each time with water daily.

e.) Ingredients:

Mong bean flour	100gm
Bai Zhi	50gm
Bai Ji	50gm
Bai Lian	50gm

Bai Jiang Can	50gm
Bai Fu Zi	50gm
Tian Hua Fen	50gm
Gan Song	25gm
Shan Nai	25gm
Mao Xiang	25gm
Ling Ling Xian	100gm
Fang Feng	100gm
Gao Ben (ligusticum sinense olive root)	
	100gm
Fei Zao Jia	two pieces.

Make all into a powder, mix, and use it to wash the face.

f.) Ingredients:

She Xiang	25gm
Zhu Yi (pork pancreas)	
	3
Man Qing Zi	150gm
peach seeds (rid of skin)	
	150gm
sheep butter	150gm.

Make into a powder and wrap the powder in a cotton cloth. Soak it in two liters of wine for three nights, sealed tightly. Apply on the face each night.

g.) For wrinkles

Pull off the thin skins of chestnuts, dry them, and make them into a fine powder. Use a little light-colored honey to make into balls. Use it as a lotion.

h.) More for wrinkles

148

Lu Jiao Shuang	100gm
cow's milk	1 liter
Bai Lian	50gm
Chuan Hong	50gm
Tian Men Dong (rid of skin, roasted)	
	75gm
butter	150 gm
Bai Zhi	50gm
Bao Fu Zi (raw)	50gm
Bai Shu	50gm
Xing Ren	50gm

Note about the Xing Ren: soak in water to remove the skin and the tip top; avoid the two-seed-in-one kind; make this separately into a fine powder. If the Xing Ren tastes bitter, it is poisonous. So don't use it. Only use those which taste good.

Make all the ingredients into a powder. Add in the Xing Ren and mix well, then put in the milk and butter. Cook at a low temperature until thick. Use as lotion every night, and rinse it off in the morning.

i.) For the skin

Beat five fresh egg whites until fluffy, then add a tablespoon of honey. Twice a week, use a soft brush to brush the mixture onto the skin; let it dry naturally, then rinse it off. If your skin is oily, you may add a teaspoon of lemon juice.

j.) For more hair

Use Jin Xing Cao, any amount as you wish. Soak it in sesame oil and apply on the head an hour before showering.

k.) For healthy hair

Huang Qi	50gm
Dang Gui	50gm
Du Huo	50gm
Chuang Hong	50gm
Bai Zhi	50gm
Shao Yao	50gm
Mang Cao	50gm
Fang Fang	50gm
Xing Yi Ren	50gm
Gan Di Huang	50gm
Gao Ben (Ligusticum sinense)	
	50gm
She Xian	50gm
Fei Bai (Allium macrostemon)	
	half liter
black sesame oil	4.5 liter
Ma She Gao	2 liters

Cook the ingredients, except the Ma She Gao, in water at low temperature until it boils three times. Wash the hair first, then use this herbal shampoo.

l.) For growing hair

Sang Ye (leaves), Ma Ye equal amounts, as much as you wish. Cook them in water and use it as shampoo. After seven days, you will see the change. Use it often, and your hair will be always nice looking and rich.

m.) For the skin

Cow's milk   250gm
fresh ginger juice
(squeezed from fresh ginger root)
                              200gm
red hot pepper powder 1/2gm
Bai Fu Ling powder   25gm
Gesin powder   25gm.

Cook the milk and ginger juice until boiling, then add in the other three ingredients. Cook it all until very thick, then make herbal balls (as big as the seed of the clerodendron tree). Take 20 balls half an hour before each meal.

n.) For the skin

Pearl powder: If you want to make it by yourself, the best kind of pearls to use should be big, shiny, and smooth. When cut in half, you will be able to see the circled lines. Wrap them in a piece of cloth and cook with a piece of tofu and water for two hours. Then rinse the pearls and add a little water. Make the powder fine, the finer the better. Then dry it into dry powder. Every ten days, take seven to eight grams with warm tea.

o.) For acne

Use raw Tu Si Zi and get the juice out of it. Put the juice on the acne area as a lotion.

3. HEALTHY WINES AND SOUPS FOR BEAUTY:

a.) Walnut (rid of skin)   400gm
   Chinese dates   200gm
   light-colored honey   200gm
   butter   100gm

apricots seeds (rid of the tip top and skin, use the single-seed kind, not the doubled-seed kind; they are a little poisonous, so cook them in water for one minute after boiled, then dry them)   50gm.

Mix honey and melted butter into a good paste first, then add the rest of the ingredients, and soak for a week. Drink three to five tablespoons in the morning daily. Sheep butter is the best because it nourishes the organs and skin, and keeps blood and channels harmonious.

b.)Dang Gui, Long Gan wine

Use an equal amount of each ingredient. Soak in good wine for three weeks; drink some daily.

c.) Bone marrow soup

Either beef, sheep, or pork bones can be used (sheep is the best) 600gm. Roast and make into a powder, add some roasted rice flour, and keep in a glass or clay jar. Take one tablespoon daily; you may take it with hot milk or water. This is not for those with high blood pressure (or overweight people). This soup nourishes the lungs and skin.

d.) Chinese date soup
   Dates   50gm

By Yanling B. Johnson

rice   90gm.
Cook together until the soup is a little thick. Drink
it often to help build up health and good looking skin.

e.) Walnut, rid of skin, ground with water into a
pulp, can be put in cooked rice soup. Eat it often.

f.) Black dry mushroom (Mu Er)
                        30gm
Chinese dates   30
Get rid of the core of the dates and make the ingre-
dients into a soup. Twice a day, eat 150 ml.

g.) He Shou Wu   25gm
Cook with rice; have the soup often.

4. FOR LOSING WEIGHT

Don't expect a sudden change – herbs, massage, and
acupuncture help you lose weight in a gentle, slow way.
The methods are not harmful, and if you use the right
one just for you, it will benefit your health, too.

a.) Tea
Tea is a natural for losing weight. Drink some hot
tea after the meal and it will help digest and cut off the
grease in the intestines.

b.) Herbal recipe
   Ingredients:
   Black and white Qian Niu Zi
                        each 10-30gm

roasted Cao Jue Ming	10 gm
Ze Xie	10gm
Bai Shu	10gm
Shan Zha	20gm
Zhi Shou Wu	20gm.

Make the above into a powder, then use some honey to make it into small balls (as big as the seed of the clerodendron tree). Take 20-30 balls twice daily, in the morning and evening.

c.) Acupuncture

Use needles in either the Liang Qiu or in the Gong Sun points, on both sides. Take turns for each treatment. The patient has to feel a strong sensation when the needles are twisted. You may connect an electronic needle for 20 minutes. Then use a skin needle on the acupoint, and leave for three days. The patient should press the hidden needle lightly two or three times, each time for one to two minutes, and press hard ten minutes before a meal or when feeling hungry. Do acupuncture every three days, ten treatments. Rest for a week, then do the second treatment. Observe the results and make a decision.

d.) Acupuncture

Choose one point at a time from San Jiao, Fei (lungs), and Nei Fen Mi points on the ears. In turns, put tiny needles in, and leave for five days. Perform six times for treatment.

e.) Acupressure

Use Wang Bu Liu Xing seeds; press them onto the points on the ear and attach tightly with a tiny bandage. The patient should feel numb, or a sore or hot feeling when pressing the seed. Each time treat only one ear, then switch to the other. Do this once a week, ten times total.

The main points are: Nei Fen Mi, Shen Men, assisted by Da Chang, Kou (mouth), Wei (stomach), Fei (lungs), and Fen Men.

f.) Acupressure

Use half mong beans. Press the beans on the points on both ears, choosing the points according to the case. For example, for endocrinopathy, use Nei Fen Mi, Qiu Nao, Luan Chao, and Nao Dian points. For eating too much, use Ji Dian, Ke Dian, spleen, and stomach points. For sleeping too much, use She Shui, Qiu Nao, and Shen Men. Each take four to six points, once a week, five times for treatment. Then rest for a week and begin the second treatment.

g.) Massage

Tui Na massage, on Zhong Fu, Yun Men, Ti Wei, Shen Wei. Press the Fu Jie, Fu She, Qi Hai, Guan Yuan points, then have the patient lie on the stomach, Tuina Pang Guang channel, press Pi Yu, Shen Yu, etc. Do this once a day, 30 times for the treatment. Some may need to rest after the treatment; then continue the second treatment.

Food That is Not Good to Eat Together

CHAPTER 19

I briefly choose some most commonly seen food in the United States. There will be another book about herbs and food, which contains the most information.

1. PLUM

Red plum can't eat with duck egg, sparrow meat. When they are eaten together it will produce poison. And plum is not good to eat with chicken, it will cause diarrhea.

Yellow color plum is not good to eat with black carp and will cause health problem.

2. CRAB

Crab is not good to eat together with pumpkin, ice, honey, raw peanuts, muskmelon, persimmon, loach (the kind of "fish" looks like snake and live in mud), eggplant, it will harm health. It is not good to eat together with orange kind either, it will cause soft kind cellulitis.

3. SNAIL

It is not good to eat with corn, muskmelon, ice, Mu Er mushroom (a Chinese vegetable), clam and will cause poison. To eat noodles with snail will cause diarrhea, and to eat it with pork will cause hair loss.

4. BEEF

Beef doesn't go with Chinese chive and it will be harmful to health.

5. MILK

Milk is not good to eat together with vinegar, it will cause intestine protuberance. Nor is it good to eat with raw fish, it will cause health problem. Nor it is good to eat with spinach, it will cause diarrhea.

6. PORK

It is not good to cook with Gan Cao (a Chinese herb) and it will be harmful to health. If you are eating pork with snail, it cause eyebrow loss.

7. SHRIMP

Don't eat shrimp with pumpkin, it may cause diarrhea.

8. LIVER

Goat liver is no good to eat with bamboo shoot and it is harmful to health.

9. CELERY

It is not good to eat with turtle meat and will cause health problems.

10. BAMBOO SHOOT

Bamboo shoot can't be eaten with malted sugar or it is harmful to your health.

Chinese Medicine Terms

CHAPTER 20

RELEASE POISON
– detoxicating or removing the poison quality of any substance

ZHONG
– the middle part of gastric cavity, stomach area

YANG QI
– denotes functional activity

YIN QI
– denotes substance as compared with yang qi, one aspect of the two opposites

CHANNEL
– passages through which qi and blood circulate

XU (QIXU, BLOOD XU, ETC.)
– a term used in many deficiency syndrome, such as debility, weakness caused by consumption

SAN JIAO
– "triple heater", including the upper - , middle - and lower (body) jiao. Their function represents the summation of the organs and also the passageways of qi and fluids

QI (CHI)
– essence of life, it flows with the water and food,

159

and the inspired air, in the blood of body fluid, etc.

REN CHANNEL
– front middle line channel

DU CHANNEL
– back middle channel

ACUPOINTS
– small pools of the circulating qi and blood of channels and viscera where acupuncture or moxibustion is applied

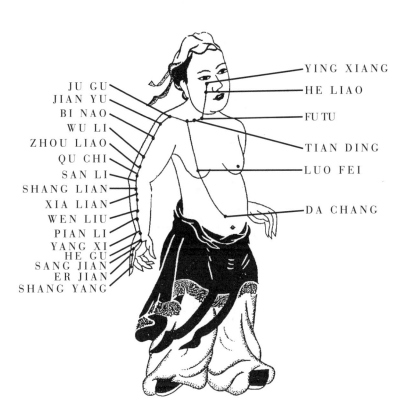

JU GU
JIAN YU
BI NAO
WU LI
ZHOU LIAO
QU CHI
SAN LI
SHANG LIAN
XIA LIAN
WEN LIU
PIAN LI
YANG XI
HE GU
SANG JIAN
ER JIAN
SHANG YANG

YING XIANG
HE LIAO
FU TU
TIAN DING
LUO FEI
DA CHANG

ANCIENT CHINESE MERIDIAN PICTURE

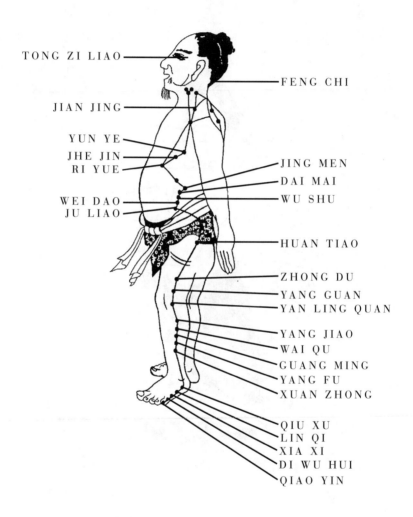

TONG ZI LIAO

FENG CHI

JIAN JING

YUN YE
JHE JIN
RI YUE

JING MEN
DAI MAI
WU SHU

WEI DAO
JU LIAO

HUAN TIAO

ZHONG DU
YANG GUAN
YAN LING QUAN

YANG JIAO
WAI QU
GUANG MING
YANG FU
XUAN ZHONG

QIU XU
LIN QI
XIA XI
DI WU HUI
QIAO YIN

ANCIENT CHINESE MERIDIAN PICTURE

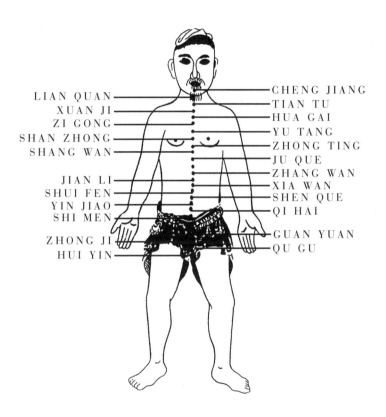

LIAN QUAN
XUAN JI
ZI GONG
SHAN ZHONG
SHANG WAN

JIAN LI
SHUI FEN
YIN JIAO
SHI MEN

ZHONG JI
HUI YIN

CHENG JIANG
TIAN TU
HUA GAI
YU TANG
ZHONG TING
JU QUE
ZHANG WAN
XIA WAN
SHEN QUE
QI HAI

GUAN YUAN
QU GU

ANCIENT CHINESE MERIDIAN PICTURE

Reference

ALL THE FOLLOWING ARE FROM THE ORIGINAL
CHINESE TEXTS.

1. Books of Dr. Nan Hui-Jin

2. Chinese Science and Qigong

3. Laozi

4. I Ching

5. Lunyu - Confucious

6. Qigong Dictionary

7. Nei Jing

8. Functional Traditional Cosmetology

9. Family Tui Na Health Care

10. Endocrinological Concepts of Chinese Qigong

11. Chinese Food Therapy Recipes

STUDY AIDS FOR SOARING CRANE QIGONG

Book: Chinese Soaring Crane Qigong by Zhao Jin-Xiang translated by Chen Hui-Xian, Pan Rui and others

Contains: Five routines
              Standing Meditation
              Remedy Routines
              Crane Walking Steps
              Questions and Answers

Video: Chinese Soaring Crane Qigong
A two-tape set of training tapes made in China by Zhao Jin-Xiang and others. They include all routines described in the book. These are training tapes, professionally done with graphics to aid in illustrating the steps. In English.

Video: Soaring Crane Practice Tape — about 1 hour long — performed by Chen Hui-Xian. This tape narrated by Chen, makes an excellent practice tape for those who have taken a class.

Audio: Five Routine Practice Audio Tape — 30 minutes per side — performed by Chen Hui-Xian. Meant to help pace you while doing the form.

Qigong Association Membership: This is a newly formed organization with Chen Hui-Xian as advisor. It is dedicated to bringing Qigong to America. It will publish a quarterly newsletter. It will be forming a strategy for continuing education and teacher certification in bringing Soaring Crane Qigong to America. The association will also be exploring other forms and aspects of Qigong.

Order Form:

Name: _____

Address: _____

City/State/ZIP: _____

Chinese Soaring Crane Qigong
(the book).................... _____ ($25 each)
Chinese Soaring Crane Qigong
(the video)................... _____ ($60 for two tapes)
Soaring Crane Practice Tape
(the video)................... _____ ($20 each)
Five Routine Audio Tape .... _____ ($5 each)
Qigong Association Membership _____ ($10 for 4 issues)
(no S&H)
Shipping and Handling
($5 for all).................. $5.00
Total .... _____

Send Check Payable to:
Qigong Association of America
27133 Forest Springs Lane
Corvallis, OR 97330

Questions? Call us at **541 745-6310**

STUDY AIDS FOR FRAGRANT QIGONG

Fragrant Qigong was introduced to the general public in 1988 by Master Tian, Rui-sheng. Since then it has become the most popular form of qigong in China with more than 90 million practitioners. It is a Buddhist form developed two thousand years ago.

The form is quite easy to learn and requires no mind work. It can be done while watching TV, walking, etc.

Chinese Fragrant Qigong - Beginning Level Video — This video, filmed in Taiwan, clearly illustrates the beginning level. The companion booklet describes the form and includes **Questions and Answers of Fragrant Qigong** by Master Tian.

Chinese Fragrant Qigong - Second Level Video — The beginning level exercises should be done for 3 to 6 months before learning the second level. There is a companion booklet further illustrating the form.

Order Form:

Name: _____

Address: _____

City/State/ZIP: _____

Chinese Fragrant Qigong
Beginning Level Video .... _____ ($25 each)
Chinese Fragrant Qigong
Second Level Video .... _____ ($25 each)
Shipping and Handling
    ($5 for all)................... $5.00
Total .... _____

Send Check Payable to:
Qigong Association of America
27133 Forest Springs Lane
Corvallis, OR 97330

Books "Herbal Food" and more Qigong books will be available in 1997.

Questions? Call us at **541 745-6310**